Endocrine

Disrupted

*exposing the dangers in
consumer products that are
making you sick*

Darlene Rose

HNC, Dipl. HHP, Cert. WC, Herb.

ISBN-10: 1523358742
ISBN-13: 978-1523358748

Acknowledgments

This book is dedicated to my husband, Richard Rose, for all the hours he left me alone to write, even though he wanted to spend time with me. For being patient with me after I asked him to read my book for the fiftieth time, because I made changes yet again. For encouraging me though he thought I could have said it better or said less. For letting me write my own book in my own style even though he has a Bachelor's degree in English.

I dedicate this book to my prophetic friends who pulled the writer out in me when I could only dream it. It is to those who reminded me that the Lord gave a word and the women published it (Psalm 68:11), and encouraged me to write the vision and make it plain (Habakkuk 2:2).

I dedicate this book to my friend Leonora Byrd, who helped me with the title, and to Kelly Dombrowski for keeping me sane through the process.

Finally, I dedicate this book to my editors, Nedra Epps of Vision Heirs Publishing and Consulting for her encouragement, hand holding and practical advice on style and structure, and to Karen Overturf, of Three Cords Publishing, for her professional advice and formatting the finished product. I felt safer having these ladies look over my work and offer such valuable insight and professional experience.

CONTENTS

Foreword

Wow! This book is a must read! Darlene has learned much of what is written here the hard way—through sickness. She has done the research for us. Some of the information contained in this book was disturbing to me; to realize that we cannot trust the safety of many products just because they are on the shelf at the store. The everyday things we have in our homes can be causing us future harm. We spend thousands of dollars on cleaners, lotions, toothpaste, deodorants, shampoos, conditioners and more, thinking they are safe. We know that obvious things like smoking can cause sickness and disease, and it is noted as such on the packaging of tobacco products; but we have been unaware that many other common household products are making us sick, and I'm shocked that very little is being done about it.

Our health depends on our own wisdom and research. We usually do not take the time unless we start getting sick, but Darlene did the work for us in assembling the information we need to know, and our part is to respond. So many people ask why God created cancer and other diseases. Guess what? God did not; man did. This book will compel you to stand up and take charge of your surroundings in your own home. It is well written, easy to understand; and it becomes clear what we need to do in order to take back our health.

Cheryl Stasinowsky, Author and Speaker
www.wordscribeministries.com

Introduction

I have a healthy body, free of the chemicals that once controlled it.
Lorna Luft

The average American household's cleaning cupboard is likely the most toxic, *UNCLEAN* cupboard in our home. There are window cleaners and all-purpose cleaners and dusting sprays and air fresheners and laundry soaps and dish soaps and floor cleaners and bug sprays and plant sprays and bleach and ammonia and bathroom scrub and mold preventers and drain uncloggers and scouring agents.

Recently, I was asked, "Do natural cleaners really work?" That is to say, "Can natural cleaning products do the same amazing job that chemically engineered products can?" My response was, "Why drop an atomic bomb inside your house when a firecracker will do?"

In our personal care closet we have antibacterial soap and antibacterial hand sanitizer and face creams and lotions and foot care and hand creams and shampoo and conditioner and hairspray and gel and shaving cream and aftershave and cheap body mists and underarm anti-perspirants and deodorants and ladies, the make-up bag? How much product do we really need? Is it really necessary?

Our refrigerator and pantry is loaded with quick, easy meals because we lead a fast-paced life. Those meals might fit within our budget, they may be tastier, they may hold promises of health and weight loss, but have you checked the ingredients? Most foods that are prepared and processed contain chemical additives you do not need in your body.

Is natural better? I am writing this book to answer that question. I had to have a better answer than, "Well, yeah."

I wanted to show why organic food is the safer choice, why natural housecleaning is the cleaner clean, and why food grade cosmetics and personal care products are more desirable and reduce your cancer risk.

But before I can answer those questions satisfactorily, I need to show you why what you are currently using is dangerous. Harmful chemicals, heavy metals and endocrine disruptors are literally making us sick!

I offer you my story. I hope you will take the information I have presented in this book to make the changes you need to make in your life in small doses. Small doses are more effective and lasting.

Darlene Rose

Chapter One

We stopped cleaning our houses with lemon water and vinegar like our mothers did, and we clean with chemicals. We're breathing chemicals, and then everyone wonders why cancer is the biggest killer.

Suzanne Somers

In the late 80's I took a part time job with a cleaning company that offered construction cleaning, as well as commercial and residential cleaning. I was exposed to many solvents, such as turpentine, mineral spirits, denatured alcohol, bleach, and ammonia to name a few. We didn't wear gloves much except on occasion. Well, I can't recall if we actually did, but I think they were available. We also did not wear masks. For a few years I breathed in the vapors of Volatile Organic Compounds (VOC's) and drywall dust and dirt. Solvents were absorbed into our skin. But when we were finished, we congratulated ourselves on a job well done. The finished product was beautiful.

I took a little time off in early 1992 due to pain in my back and stomach. When I lay down it felt like I was laying on a grapefruit. After a visit to the doctor, I learned I had a rapidly growing tumor on my uterus. X-rays then revealed that it was so attached to the uterus that both the uterus and right ovary would need to be removed. I had a partial hysterectomy in March 1992.

After recovery, I looked into gaining my own

customers and eventually did residential cleaning only. While I enjoyed the money of construction and commercial cleaning, I enjoyed even more the relationship I had with my own customers who also loved the way I cleaned. I found some great ways to make a house shine with lemon oil (not lemon ESSENTIAL oil (*Citrus limon*), but lemon oil, such as in Old English Lemon Oil – there is a difference). I used it on everything from PVC outdoor patio furniture to the chrome on sinks and stoves (to my dismay often leaving a trail of oil behind, but that was my creative learning curve).

By 1994 I had some disturbing symptoms. Something was very wrong with me that I could not describe well at all. Depression was settling in, and I was sad without apparent reason. I experienced uncontrollable emotions, and friends closest to me suggested I see a counselor. I didn't need one, I reasoned, because my sadness was not due to a traumatic life event. I insisted what I was feeling was very, very physical, yet could not describe the feeling. I thought that perhaps I was experiencing menopause since I had a hysterectomy a few years prior. After seeing the endocrinologist, she told me I was not in menopause, that my left ovary was producing enough estrogen for my body's needs. She did, however, prescribe an estrogen patch to see if I felt better.

Six months later I was scheduled for a breast exam with my gynecologist. The morning of my appointment, I woke up with intense pain in my right breast. Even the air caused it pain. I called to see if I could get an earlier time because I thought something was terribly wrong, and they took me right away. The doctor noticed a red line going from my nipple to my underarm. The office went into crisis response mode. I didn't know what was happening until I saw the needle that was probably 6 inches long, yet looked and felt like 10 feet. He said, "You have a red streak." The doctor found a lump and biopsied it, then told me it was situated in an area of my breast that was blocking a duct. He scheduled surgery for me to have the lump removed. I was thankful it was benign but I learned that it could have been triggered by the estrogen patch.

I experienced a disabling fatigue that I had not known before. Rest. Rest. Rest was all I needed, and if I could just get more rest I'd feel better. But that feeling of relief did not come even though I could sleep up to 18 hours per day, often calling into work, unable to go. I felt pain and stiffness in my muscles and joints. My movement was very limited. I took OTC Motrin (OTC Motrin is 200 mg per tablet of ibuprofen, but prescription-strength Motrin is 800 mg). I took the equivalent of about 4 prescription- strength Motrin a day to find relief (I later learned that this was toxic to my liver). I recall feeling like I was having a heart attack. I could describe this pain as my chest or stomach muscles contracting, taking my breath away. I went to a walk-in clinic where I was diagnosed with Costochondritis (inflammation of the cartilage that connects the rib to the breast bone). The suggested course of action was to take some ibuprofen, but I was already taking more than I should have. It didn't make sense to me.

For a season, I recall lying in bed, unable to get out of bed. My brain was telling my right arm to move but it was as if it were stuck to the bed. I had to take my left arm, grab my right arm, pick it up and roll over onto my left side, then roll off the bed. I would crawl on the floor to the bathroom and then to the bathtub. Once there, I found relief by turning on the cold water and running my hands under it. When that relief came, I would place my hands on the tub to lift myself up and then move to the sink. From there, I could splash cold water on my face and arms. I did not know why it was cold water that relieved me until years later when I learned that my body was *inflamed* and the cold water was healing to me.

I had to quit the cleaning business because it was too physical for me at that time. I had been experiencing internal tremors, in addition to the pain, which were not visible to anyone but me. I did not know that chemicals, endocrine-disrupting chemicals, and neurotoxins, were affecting me. I saw several doctors for the pain and fatigue, but all they offered me were various anti-depressants that did not help much. I was, however, less emotional. That translated into experiencing less of ALL emotions, including laughter, joy, and excitement. I was unable to be hugged, held, or rubbed up against without pain but had become able, finally, to describe how I felt. I was a walking bruise but no longer cried about it.

When I was able to describe the pain, a doctor diagnosed me in 1995 as having fibromyalgia. Back then, very little was known about fibromyalgia. When you break down the word, it means Fibrous Muscle Pain. I thought, "How is this a diagnosis? What causes it?" If I was able to find a doctor who would agree with the diagnosis, I might be able to get some questions answered and perhaps treatment, but I was unable. The doctor who diagnosed me was out of my insurance network and quite a distance away. He could make the diagnosis, but could only offer me anti-depressants to help ease the pain.

The internet was not widely available at the time, and we did not have a computer for me to look it up. I was unable to find a book at the library on it, so I turned to the Lord. I did not know what caused fibromyalgia, but I did find some relief through meditation.

I learned to overcome stress by meditating on God's word and waiting for Him to speak to my soul. Stress, whether emotional, physical or external, triggered something in my body causing it to flare up. Over the next few years I learned how to overcome stress. I learned forgiveness. I learned I didn't have to be overcome by this, but could overcome all things through Christ who strengthens me. I learned I can do all things, just not all at once.

I also learned the word "toxic"—toxic behaviors, toxic relationships, toxic emotions, and toxic chemicals. These all caused flare-ups (note the words *flare up* refer to fire inside the body or *inflammation*).

I had a reaction to foods that caused inflammation— wheat, liquid dairy (milk as opposed to cheese), etc. I started to wean myself off these products, not giving them up entirely, because I seemed to be okay eating small amounts.

My belly would bloat. I'd watch it rise like a basketball before my eyes. My clothing had to be loose-fitting because my belly could bloat after eating or after stress. I'd close my eyes and picture water filling the empty spaces in my gut and displacing the air or gas that caused it to rise. *"But why does it rise so much?"* I meditated.

I was unable to be touched. I kept others at arm's length from me because it hurt me even as someone brushed past me. I could not be hugged. My husband was afraid that every time he came near me he would put me in pain. How could you give up hugs? I had to.

In March 2005, I quit a 33-year smoking habit. Within 3 weeks of being smoke free, I felt a burning sensation, accompanied by internal tremors in my body that no doctor could diagnose. The burning sensation was excruciating, and I felt like a blow torch was hitting it. I did not realize at that time that I was possibly experiencing the neurotoxins from the cigarettes after quitting. This time, only heat would remedy it. Cold air was agony. Fortunately, I lived in Florida. But unfortunately, most places needed to be air-conditioned.

I saw several doctors, but they were puzzled. One doctor sent me to a neurologist who could not find anything wrong, then sent me to another neurologist who ordered an MRI. The MRI revealed nothing. It was suggested I go back on anti-depressants. I refused. I knew something was wrong, and anti-depressants only masked whatever it was. I went to work wearing blazers and covered my face as much as I could. I requested being away from the air-conditioner (imagine living in Florida during the hot summer months and wearing jackets in the office). Spending hours in the sun helped. In fact, any warmth helped. When driving alone, the air-conditioner had to be off and windows cracked only slightly in order to breathe, while the temperature rose to sometimes 90 degrees or more. Apparently cold water relieved the inflammation inside my body, while the heat of the air was necessary to relieve the pain in my nerves.

By spring 2006, my husband was offered a position in West Virginia. Most people who understood my "condition" thought it was crazy for me to go because of my being unable to handle cold air temperatures.

Chapter Two

How is it that mercury is not safe for food additives and over the Counter drug products, but it is safe in our vaccines and dental amalgams?

Dan Burton

The first summer in Charleston, West Virginia I felt great. The temperature of the air was right, and I did not find a job right away, so was not exposed to many chemicals from offices and air conditioners. Our apartment did not have central air, but we had a window unit and I kept it off as much as possible. By the time it started getting colder, I could feel pain in my face, my fingers, and my legs. The tremors returned with a vengeance. By winter 2007, I thought I was dying. I described this pain as a "river of poison" running through my body.

Little did I know that the locals had a nickname for Charleston: "Chemical Valley." I learned there were more than 30 chemical companies including Dow, Union Carbide, and Bayer Crop Science right here in Kanawha County. Some had closed down by this time, but even the locals would laugh that snow never sticks in Charleston due to the heat from the chemicals that were put out.

I drove by the Healing Rooms of Charleston and, eventually, started to attend the church where the Director of the Healing Rooms attended. I decided to go there for prayer.

There was a team of three people praying for someone else, so I waited in the lobby until I was called, "Mrs. Rose, you can come in now." Mike Parsons, who led the team, prayed over me that day. I walked into a little room with a few chairs against the wall and one in the center of the room. "Please have a seat here," Mike offered. "How can we pray for you today?"

I shared my history of pain, fatigue, tremors and no relief, no real help. He and the others began to pray. A few minutes into the prayer, Mike paused. "I'm smelling gum. Does that mean anything to you?" he asked.

"No." I responded. So he started praying again, then paused. "I'm smelling it strongly. It's like cinnamon. In fact, it's like that gum that was advertised when we were kids. It had like a red packaging."

"Clark's Teaberry Gum?" I asked.

"Yes! That's it! Does that mean anything to you?" he asked.

"No, it does not. I don't chew gum." I responded again.

Mike and the team continued praying. He stopped the prayer and said "The Lord is telling me to tell you 'Get the gum and chew on it.'"

Any other person may have thought this was hokey, but I knew in my spirit that this was from the Lord. I did not know why or what it meant, but I sensed there was something to this.

I left the Healing Rooms to get into the car then thought, "Clarks' Teaberry gum? Where would I ever find that? Was it still on the market?" Nonetheless, I spoke aloud, while driving, "Lord, if this was a word from You, lead me to where I would find Clark's Teaberry Gum."

I started down the road and found Foodland. "Okay, I'll check there." As soon as I walked through the entrance doors, there was a gum stand with Clark's Teaberry gum on it facing me. By this time, I was certain this was a word from God. I bought the gum. Once inside the car I opened it up and started chewing on it. "Okay Lord, I'm chewing on it."

I hated gum. Once, I chewed gum and it stuck to my fillings and pulled a little filling out. My mind wandered to a story of a miracle that was told to me the previous day in which the attendees of a healing conference found their silver fillings were replaced with gold. All of a sudden, I had an AHA moment! God was removing fillings in that conference because they were asking for healing! My symptoms? Could they be, at least in part, from fillings?

I threw the gum out and drove home on a mission. I ran into the house, up the stairs, turned on the computer and started to look up mercury fillings. I found that mercury toxicity could be behind all the symptoms I was experiencing for years. (1) (3)

But why Clark's Teaberry Gum? Was there a significance there? I believe that, because I recognized the gum from my childhood, my toxic symptoms originated from childhood.

I found a dentist who would remove and replace my fillings, a mercury-free dentist, actually. I had eight fillings, but we could only remove two at a time. When the dentist drills a filling, the particles are more easily absorbed into the saliva and then carried into the bloodstream, therefore I had what looked like a dryer vent hooked up to my mouth to capture the particles and properly dispose them. She and her staff were covered from head to toe with protective clothing to shield them from mercury particles that didn't get sucked up into this vent. After two filling removals, I then went over to have chelation therapy at a nearby holistic clinic. There, I would receive an IV of 50,000 IU's of Vitamin C for 3 hours as it flushed all the toxins out of my body. I did this 4 times. But before I began chelation therapy, I had a test for heavy metals toxicity. Sure enough, mercury was in the red zone. Tin was off the charts. The doctor told me that he was confident I was toxic due to the fillings in my teeth as opposed to eating fish because of the tin that was present. In fact, there is, actually, a small amount of silver in the amalgam mixture. Fillings are 50% mercury, and the remainder is a combination of silver, tin and copper.

By the second treatment I was already feeling better than I had in over a decade. Color flooded my face again, and I no longer trembled. I could handle the cold and the heat. I was not depressed. I had more energy than I could remember ever having.

My conversations with the administering physician, Dr. John McCallum, were regarding toxicity, heavy metals, chemicals, etc. I asked him about my cleaning supplies. Could they also have contributed to this? Yes, indeed. Most toxins are filtered out by the liver; but if the liver is already damaged or injured by toxicity, it will not be able to do its job well, and toxins will continue to build up in our bodies.

I already knew I had an enlarged liver. I had a 13-year drug and alcohol addiction that began in the early 1970s. My liver became enlarged and sluggish. Once I was clean and sober, I thought that was enough. Looking back, it became clear that my liver was unable to filter out additional toxins that came from processed foods, water, and environment, let alone the heavy metals. I was always fighting symptoms.

According to Stephen B. Edelson, MD, an estimated twenty-five percent of the population have some form of heavy metal poisoning. Studies have shown that exposure to toxic metals such as mercury, cadmium, lead, arsenic, aluminum, nickel and other heavy metals can be linked to the autoimmune process. (43)The heavy metals may induce autoimmune diseases by triggering the production of autoantibodies, antibodies that attack the body's own proteins. Chronic fatigue syndrome, fibromyalgia, lupus, Sjogren's, rheumatoid arthritis, Raynaud's, rosacea, myasthenia gravis, Hashimoto's, type 2 diabetes, multiple sclerosis have all been triggered by constant toxic stress. Mercury directly damages our tissues, making them look foreign to the immune system. (4) To prevent the harmful effects of heavy metals on the immune system, it is crucial to assess your potential toxin exposure, understand where the source of the toxins originated, and take as many steps as possible to remove these toxins from your body and your environment.

Chapter Three

God doesn't just miraculously and physically intervene in the whole process, so if I just go and drop a bunch of chemicals and herbicides that leach into the groundwater, I can pray all day to keep my child healthy, but if the herbicides gone into the groundwater come up my well, my child's going to drink that water.

Joe Salatin

"Aquapocolypse" was the nickname being given to the chemical spill into the Elk River in West Virginia which managed to disrupt the lives of over 300,000 people in 9 counties and temporarily shut down businesses, schools, hospitals, daycares, restaurants and any other operation that carried a permit to serve food and drink. The chemical, 4-methylcyclohexanemethanol, or MCHM, leaked to the Elk River from a defective storage tank on January 9, 2014.

The smell of licorice permeated the air in downtown Charleston at about 10 a.m., but some started smelling it about 7 a.m. on their way to work. At the time, it was unclear as to the origin of the smell, but by noon the social media was abuzz.

I learned of the *Do Not Use* order later on for Kanawha County, and four other counties at 5:30 p.m., when I turned the television on to watch the news. By 9:00 that evening the ban had expanded to nine counties. This order prohibited the use of tap water for bathing, cooking, drinking, and laundering. We were not even to inhale it. Boiling the water did no good. In fact, the steam would produce a vapor which would intensify the chemical's effect.

Governor Earl Ray Tomblin declared a state of emergency. The leak, which was first reported at 11:40 a.m., came from a 48,000 gallon storage tank owned by Freedom Industries, which sits right on the river about a mile upstream from the American Water Treatment Facility. "All we know is that they discovered a hole in the tank, and material was leaking," Tom Aluise, a spokesman for the West Virginia environmental department, said. "How that hole got there, we don't know." Aluise added, "The biggest worry from the substance was if people drank it. This material pretty much floats on the water, and it's floating downstream, and eventually it will dissipate, but you can't actually get in there and remove it." (5) The leaked product is used in the froth flotation process of coal washing and preparation. It initially leaked into a containment area, and the product then leaked from the containment area into the river.

Everyone scurried into grocery stores and retail outlets, as well as convenience stores. Anyplace that sold bottled water was packed within a few hours. Water, baby wipes, paper plates, cups and utensils were soon off the shelves. By the next morning, lines of people formed at all stores as they waited for the next shipment of bottled water to arrive. The chaos intensified. Fear and anger gripped many as they waited also for answers to when this would be over. Some had their carts snatched from them like thieves snatched a purse. Social media lit up with outrage; people started arguing over who was to blame and hateful language spewed out towards each other as well as towards Gary Southern, Executive of Freedom Industries, and West Virginia American Water. Class Action lawsuits had begun.

This chemical was virtually unknown. There were no safety procedures in place for any leakage. The Centers for Disease Control had to give it their most educated guess at coming up with a safety standard of 1 part per million.

West Virginia was now known all over the world within a day. It drew the attention of Erin Brokovich, who at the time I began writing some of the details of this book, was in town with her investigative team. Most counties had their ban lifted by day 9 of the crisis and had begun or finished the process of flushing out their tanks in order to have potable water again.

Many residents continued to smell licorice after the ban lifted. Some had gotten headaches. Some complained of nausea. Some reported burns. Others had difficulty breathing. Although my husband and I were living in the red zone, we were among the very few that were symptom free. According to the health department, 411 patients were treated at hospitals for symptoms that were attributed to exposure to the chemical, and 20 people were admitted. Also, more than 1,600 people called poison control to complain of symptoms.

Karen Bowling, West Virginia's Secretary of Health and Human Resources said the department was trying to sort out how many of those patients were actually sickened by the chemical, and not by other diseases. (6)

West Virginians were angry. They were angry because their safety was not considered above profit; angry because there were no safety inspections at this chemical storage facility since 1991; angry because this storage facility was located a little over a mile upstream from the city's water treatment facility.

We know the company responsible for the chemical spill. Freedom Industries has filed for bankruptcy. This company bought the facility just two weeks prior to the spill and faced nine lawsuits.

But what if we didn't know anything about the company? What if we knew of no one to blame for exposing us to toxic chemicals and poisoning our water? What if, no single company was involved? What if, it was us?

Chapter Four

Government and other scientists have identified hundreds of chemicals that are linked to diseases in small concentrations and that are unregulated in drinking water or policed at limits that still pose serious risks.

Charles Duhigg

In the headwaters of the Potomac River scientists have discovered that male small-mouthed bass were producing eggs. The West Virginia Division of Natural Resources asked the US Geological Survey to examine the fish near the town of Moorfield, about three hours from Washington D.C. after learning about fish die-offs in the South Potomac in 2002. Anglers reported fish with lesions. It was determined by the USGS these fish were exposed to bacteria and other contaminants.

Another test was conducted a year later, and it revealed that male fish had testicular and ovarian tissue. Some 42 percent of male small-mouth bass surveyed showed signs of inter-sex development. A second sampling produced an even higher rate—79 percent showed sexual abnormalities, according to Leetown Science Center in Kearneysville, WV. (7)

The cause of intersex development in fish has been debated, but under suspicion are emerging contaminants known as endocrine disruptors (ED's). ED's work like biological disinformation campaigns, potentially affecting any system in the body that is controlled by hormones. Sometimes mimicking natural hormones like estrogen, ED's can alter other hormone concentrations, interfering with the normal cell-signaling process by turning on, shutting off, or disrupting the signals that hormones carry. (7)

Sexual abnormalities are not confined to West Virginia waters. David O. Norris, a professor in the University of Colorado's Department of Integrative Physiology, has specialized in environmental endocrinology for over 35 years. He was involved in leading an ongoing research project which looked into hormone production in the Denver waters. He studied fish that were located below and above sewage treatment plants where effluents are added to the waters, and found reproductive abnormalities in fish downstream of the treatment plants. His impression was that the male fish were being feminized because of the contaminants in the water, mostly estrogenic. Some of the chemicals he found in the waters were estrogenic compounds from human urine originating from birth control pills. He also found large concentrations of chemicals from household detergents and personal care products. (8)

Experts on endocrine disruptors have become increasingly concerned over the presence of contaminants in drinking water. Robert W. Masters of the National Ground Water Association, NGWA (Pharmaceuticals and Endocrine Disruptors in Rivers and on Tap, 2011) raised concerns about the public water system after it had tested positive for drugs. He wrote in his article that tap water in Wheeling, WV and the Ohio River tested positive for antibiotics, according to USA TODAY, November 7, 2000. (9)

The NGWA conference held in Minneapolis, June 7, 2000, was covered on Minnesota Public Radio on "Morning Edition" June 8. Keynote Speaker Janet Raloff, author of "Drugged Waters," and Dana Kolpin of the U.S. Geological Survey were interviewed. Pharmaceuticals and endocrine disrupting chemicals in water sparked international interest as scientists from the United States, Canada, England, and Germany attended the ground-breaking conference at the Hyatt Regency, Minneapolis. Large-scale investigations were being done in over 100 of America's rivers and streams. Current drinking water standards do not require testing for any of the over 7,000 pharmaceutical compounds being prescribed.

Normal functions of all organ systems are regulated by endocrine factors. Small disturbances in endocrine function, especially during certain stages of the life cycle, can lead to profound and lasting effects. There is evidence that invertebrates, fish, avian, reptilian, and mammalian species have been adversely affected by exposure to environmental contaminants that effect the endocrine systems. (Masters, 2011) The endocrine system excretes hormones in an organism that govern many functions, including sexual and reproductive characteristics. Agricultural, industrial, and household products often contain compounds that mimic estrogen when ingested. ED's of this type may contribute to the high percentage of male small-mouth bass found in the Potomac that exhibit female characteristics.

ED's are found in many of the everyday products we use, such as household cleaning products, plastic bottles, food can liners, cosmetics and pesticides. These hormones and hormone-like substances are typically highly soluble in water and are easily transported in the blood. They are of particular concern because they can alter the critical hormonal balances required for proper health and development. The glands that make up the endocrine system are the adrenal glands, pancreas, ovaries, testes, pineal gland and the thymus, all of which are potentially affected by endocrine disruptors. (10)

Studying the fish in rivers and streams is a way to track ecological changes and learn the potential health impact on humans. According to Vicki Blazer, a scientist at Leetown Science Center, "The water resources division of USGS out of Charleston put out what are called "passive samplers" at a number of the sites." She said, "Basically they accumulate contaminants that fish tissue would accumulate over time." She and the team have been able to get a better idea of what chemicals are present that may be affecting local fish populations. Of the 161 target chemicals measured in the five passive-water samples, 100 (62%) were found in a least one such sample. The chemicals detected included 29 industrial/commercial chemicals, 24 insecticides, 20 prescription/nonprescription pharmaceuticals, 10 household/personal care products, six biogenic hormones/sterols, five herbicides, three natural fragrances, two flame retardants, and 1 fungicide. There were 25 chemicals that were found at all five sites where passive samplers were deployed. (45)

According to Blazer, almost all of our knowledge about concentrations likely to cause health concerns are based on acute toxicity or gross impacts such as changes in size. Most often there are no criteria for effects that fall below lethal, such as immune modulation or endocrine disruption. Methods used in past studies may not have been sensitive enough to detect the concentration of contaminants thought to affect the fish.

In a study of female bass from the Shenandoah River, South Fork scientists found that BDE (a flame retardant), Triclosan (an antibacterial and antifungal agent used in a wide variety of consumer products including toothpaste, mouthwash, deodorant and cleaning supplies) and pesticides had accumulated selectively within the endocrine systems of fish with lower concentrations in the brain, skin, and kidneys. (They did not accumulate in the muscle, so fortunately the fish can still be eaten.) (10)

ED's can sometimes affect reproduction, development, and behavior in organisms. Potentially, endocrine-disrupting chemicals come from a variety of sources and have diverse molecular structures.

If these chemicals are introduced into water systems from human waste and food, then it is possible that human tissues might also contain detectable levels of contaminants. We may, for example, be experiencing subtle population changes from chemical exposure that are particularly impactful during fetal and newborn development. Other known possible effects on humans caused by chemical contaminants in tissues of the endocrine system include: cancer (particularly breast cancer and testicular cancer), infertility, disorders of sex development, asthma and other immune related syndromes; autism, ADHD, learning and behavioral disorders; diabetes, thyroid disorders, poor semen quality, testes cancer, undescended testes and hypospadias, a condition in which the opening of the urethra is on the underside of the penis. (10)

In a statement made by Linda S. Birnbaum, (Director of the National Institute of Environmental Health Sciences) on February 25, 2010 before the Committee on Energy and Commerce, Subcommittee on Energy and the Environment at the US House of Representatives, there are four aspects of exposure to endocrine disruptors which need emphasis.

> • *First, the effect of low doses. Normal endocrine signaling involves very small changes in hormone levels, yet these changes can have significant biological effects. That means subtle disruptions of endocrine signaling is a plausible mechanism by which chemical exposures at low doses can have effects on the body.*

> • *Second, the wide range of effects. Endocrine signals govern virtually every organ and process in the body. That means that when outside chemicals interfere with those systems, the effects can be seen in many different diseases and conditions – some of which we are just learning to recognize as the result of endocrine disruption.*

> • *Third, the persistence of effects. We are finding that the effects of exposure to endocrine disruptors can be observed long after the actual exposure has ceased. This is*

especially true for growth and development, processes that are very sensitive to endocrine regulation. The question of how these kinds of latent effects occur is an active area of investigation.

*• **Fourth, the ubiquity of exposure.** Both naturally occurring and man-made substances can be endocrine disruptors. Some, e.g., arsenic and agricultural chemicals, are ubiquitous in the environment. In addition to the growing use of hormonally-active pharmaceuticals that pass through the bodies of those taking them and end up in water treatment systems and surface waters, many of the chemicals that are being found to have endocrine effects are components of a wide range of consumer products, including some water bottles, cosmetics, sunscreens, and other personal care products. Substances applied to the skin can be directly absorbed but also end up getting washed off our bodies and into our water systems. As a result, chemicals with endocrine disrupting activity are widely dispersed in our environment, often at levels plausibly associated with biological effects; exposure to humans is widespread.* (11)

Research on ED's is ongoing and studies may need to be conducted over many years before we have a clear picture of the challenge these present environmental issues, specifically in our drinking water supply, have on local populations. Until those studies are conclusive we don't have to be powerless. Let's take a look at what we have power over right now, in our own household environment. Our cabinets and cupboards hold a large number of household cleaning and personal care products. Have you ever considered their toxic effects?

Chapter Five

Chemicals are not currently tested for their endocrine disruption potential before they are approved for use and enter our environment, and there are endocrine disruptors in a vast array of products we come into contact with every day, including organochlorine pesticides, plastics, fuels, and other industrial chemicals.

Joel Fuhrman

Volatile Organic Compounds (VOC's) are a large group of organic compounds that can easily evaporate at room temperature. Sometimes odor can be detected but odor is not an indicator of level of risk. There are thousands of VOC's produced and used in our daily lives but here are just a few examples:

Acetone

Benzene

Ethylene glycol

Formaldehyde

Methylene chloride

Perchloroethylene

Toluene

Xylene

1,3-butadiene

VOCs refer to a group of chemicals. Each chemical has its own toxicity and potential for causing different health effects, such as, on a low level, eye, nose and throat irritation, headaches, and asthma to, on a higher level, cancer, liver, kidney or central nervous system damage. Among the sources of VOC's are household products such as cleaners, detergents, paint, carpeting and cosmetics. Studies have shown that the level of indoor VOC's is generally two to five times higher than that of outdoor VOC's.

The Minnesota Department of Health's website states the best health protection measure is to limit your exposure to products and materials that contain VOCs when possible. If you think you may be having health problems caused by VOCs, try reducing levels in your home. If symptoms persist, consult with your doctor to rule out other serious health conditions that may have similar symptoms.

A 15-year study concluded that women who work in the home are at a 54% higher risk of developing cancer than women who work outside the home, whether in another building or outdoors. (12) Homes built since 1990 were more air efficient. Windows were sealed tighter keeping outdoor air out, and central air conditioning was becoming the normal feature in a newly built home, rather than an additional option. The problem I saw with this is that while we were getting better at keeping toxic outdoor air out, we were also getting better at creating an indoor environment that allows for the buildup of VOC's in the home with no place to escape. Sometimes it's just wise to open the windows and do some air exchanging.

Approximately 70,000 chemicals are now in commercial production, many of which are used in household products. Residues of more than 400 toxic chemicals have been identified in human blood and fat tissue. (13) They accumulate in the human body, causing cancer and other diseases, yet they have been inadequately tested or remain completely untested for their safety.

Labeling laws are not adequately designed to protect the consumer, instead they are marketing banners designed to sell products and downplay real risks. The New York Poison Control Center reports that 85% of product warning labels are to assist in properly and quickly identifying a poison, (in poisoning cases, time is critical) and for first aid instructions only. Formaldehyde, phenol, benzene, toluene, and xylene are found in common household cleaners, cosmetics, beverages, fabrics and cigarette smoke. These chemicals are cancer causing and toxic to the immune system, yet are not commonly included on labels of the products in which they occur.

When using chlorine bleach or antiseptics in industrial areas it is required to wear impermeable protective clothing, hard hats, boots, gloves, apron or coveralls, chemical goggles or full-face shield and use in well ventilated areas. In the workplace, it is required to have posted warnings about toxic chemical use. In the home, there is no such requirement yet many of the same chemicals are in our cupboards and cabinets. If there was such a law, what homemaker would take the time to wear this type of protective clothing and who would regulate it? Wouldn't it be easier to reduce the use of toxic chemicals in the home? The Cancer Prevention Coalition has published a Cancer Prevention Alert listing the hazardous ingredients in household products as these products are not under any obligation to list ingredients on their labels. (13)

I looked into some of the "green cleaners" on the market today. When something is labeled as "green" it is generally considered by the public to be safe, non-toxic, and all-natural. However,

"…most cleaning products on the market are toxic chemical cocktails, and when you spritz your bathtub or kitchen counter with that brightly colored liquid you're exposing yourself and your family to endocrine-disrupting phthalates such as carcinogenic benzene, and organ-damaging phenols, just to name a few." (14)

It is quite common for commercial "green" cleaners to be toxic; the only thing "green" about them is their color and perhaps their name. Dr. Mercola, a leading authority on health, nutrition and wellness, has looked into the ingredients in many products, such as Simple Green, and states they are toxic. Several products contain 4% 2-Butoxyethanol by volume, according to the Material Safety Data Sheet (MSDS) on household products, (15) which is linked to at least 10 different diseases including liver cancer and osteoarthritis. It is a petrochemical solvent that is known to destroy red blood cells and cause minor birth defects and reproductive problems. 2-Butoxyethanol is banned in the UK. As previously noted, one of the most disturbing things is that the more "air efficient" a home is, the less opportunity that chemical buildup from products in the home can escape. People spend 90% of their time indoors. According to Mercola,

"In the case of the very young, such as infants, whose blood-brain barrier and detoxification systems are not yet fully developed, the danger may be hundreds of times higher than for adults." (14)

Cleaning products that have the label "Eco-friendly" or "Green" or "All-Natural" are not necessarily free from hazardous chemicals. These are words cleverly used for marketing purposes, and the manufacturers know they do not need to back them up with an ingredients label.

Dr. Mercola does endorse products such as Seventh Generation, Ecover, Mrs. Meyer's, Sun & Earth, as well as Orange Plus. They are more expensive, but they are concentrated and safer to use.

Chapter Six

I entered the cosmetics industry because I wanted more women to use cosmetics made with safe, healthful ingredients.

Gloria Swanson

I have seen many bathroom countertops and cabinets since 1989 when I first started cleaning homes. Most of them were filled with everything from shampoos and conditioners to soaps and face creams and deodorants and anti-perspirants and perfumes–to name just a few.

Most people tend to overlook the fact that what they put on their skin can be just as toxic as what they put into their mouths. In fact, some even more so. According to Ruth Winter, MS, in her book "A Consumer's Guide to Cosmetic Ingredients," some products are excellent but a lot of compounds in other products do nothing and are fraudulent in their claims because they contain toxins and cancer-causing agents." (16)

You might be wondering why the FDA doesn't protect us. Cosmetics have been a low priority at the FDA and its regulatory powers so weakened they are virtually non-existent. It once was assumed that the skin is impermeable and prevents toxins from entrance to the body but we now know this to be incorrect. Even cosmetic companies know that an increasingly popular way to deliver drugs is transdermally. There is the estrogen patch, the birth control patch, the pain patch, and the nicotine patch, to name a few. If these patches, when placed on the skin, can deliver the medicine necessary to effectively treat a patient, why would we think that putting a lotion on the skin would keep some of the toxic chemicals that are in that product out?

So, why IS the FDA so powerless? The Report of the Subcommittee on Science and Technology on the FDA Science and Mission at Risk gave some answers. First, the FDA's scientific organizational structure is weak. It cannot fulfill its mission because its scientific workforce does not have sufficient capacity and capability and its information technology (IT) infrastructure is inadequate. No matter how skilled and well-intentioned the FDA may be, they are crushed under an impossible workload. Some cosmetic companies will voluntarily make their safety data available and forward their information to the FDA. Only an estimated 35-40% of companies actually do. (17)

Meanwhile, it's up to the consumer to do the research. Trade organizations, such as the Personal Care Products Council (PCPC), are doing a brilliant job of establishing its own safety assessment system, the Cosmetic Ingredient Review (CIR). Since its origin in 1976, CIR panels have reviewed 1,298 ingredients as of August 2006. Of that number:

- 781 ingredients were found safe

- 408 ingredients were considered safe with qualifications

- 119 ingredients could not be evaluated due to insufficient data

- 9 ingredients were unsafe (18)

The Environmental Working Group (EWG) has created a database for consumers to understand what is in cosmetics. As of September 15, 2015, the EWG has been reviewing a new chemical, called triphenyl phosphate, which has been found in nail polish and has a potential to disrupt the endocrine system and cause obesity. Findings are yet to be reported but you can check back on their website, *Skin Deep*, periodically. (44) You can also download the free mobile app of the same name to use while you are shopping.

One of the most difficult issues in the identification of ingredients and contaminants in cosmetics is that of cancer causing ingredients. An investigative branch of Congress, called the General Accounting Office (GAO) has identified more than 125 cosmetic ingredients suspected of causing cancer as well as birth defects. Nearly all chemicals known to be carcinogenic have been shown to be mutagenic but not all mutagens are carcinogenic. This would explain why animal studies were necessary. Chemicals that cause cancer in lab mice and rats may possibly cause cancer in humans.

Two contaminants found in cosmetics have been shown to cause cancer. One is n-nitrosodiethanolamine (NDELA), which penetrates easily through the skin when used in a fatty base. NDELA is a contaminant produced when two otherwise safe ingredients are combined: amines (surfactants, emulsifiers, and detergents) and nitrites (such as in the preservative 2-bromo-2-nitropane-1,3 diol (BNDP)). The other is a 1,4-dioxane, a contaminant of raw materials. About one-third of the emulsion-based cosmetics containing polyoxyethylene derivatives contain amounts of 1,4-dioxane ranging from 1 to 25 percent.

Experts in the field of safety say that consumers do not read the labels on cosmetics, let alone warning labels. It is extremely important to not only read what is in your cosmetics, but understand what each of these ingredients are. Winter does a phenomenal job in listing these ingredients and their function in a product, as well as their danger.

Of varying concern is the anti-perspirant. Winter defines anti-perspirant as any substance having a mild astringent action that tends to reduce the size of the pores and thus restrain the passage of moisture on local body areas. The most commonly used anti-perspirant compound is aluminum chlorohydrate. Zirconium compounds are found in creams but have been discontinued as a compound in anti-perspirants because of their suspected carcinogens. The FDA has classified anti-perspirants as drugs, rather than cosmetics.

Scientists agree that aluminum-based anti-perspirants can block the ducts that allow for the sweat to be released in the armpit, prohibiting the release of toxins. They also agree that there are compounds in these products that mimic estrogen. Estrogen and estrogen mimickers and disruptors increase the potential for breast cancer cells to grow and since the armpit is close to the breast, the use of anti-perspirants is advised against by many health advocates. Clinical studies showing a remarkably high incidence of breast cancer in the upper outer quadrant of the breast together with reports of genomic instability in outer quadrants of the breast provide supporting evidence for a role for locally applied cosmetic chemicals in the development of breast cancer. (19) Deodorants do not share the same reputation as antiperspirants. Deodorants help kill the bacteria that produce odor but do not block the ducts preventing perspiration.

Of greater concern are parabens, preservatives shown to have estrogen disrupting (ED) activity. Parabens tend to build up in breast tissue. A 2004 study found parabens in 18 out of 20 samples of tissue from breast tumors. (20)

Winter defines parabens as a preservative commonly used in about 75-90 percent of cosmetics, with water being the only ingredient more commonly used. They have an antibacterial and antimicrobial activity and were believed to be safe for human use. However, in a study published in 2004 in the Journal of Applied Toxicology, it is reported that parabens are indeed a cause for concern. Traces of parabens were found by British researchers in twenty women who had breast tumors. They act like estrogen and can cause some woman to get cancer. There are plenty of paraben-free cosmetics on the market. Ingredients such as oats, pomegranate, pineapples and ginger are being substituted.

About 1 out of every 8 ingredients among the 82,000 ingredients available in our personal care products are chemicals including carcinogens, pesticides, reproductive toxins, and ED's.

Here is a list of toxic chemicals to be aware of:

- BHA & BHT
- Coal tar dyes: p-phenylenediamine and colors listed as "CI" followed by a five digit number
- DEA-related products
- Di-butyl phthalate
- Formaldehyde-releasing preservatives
- Parabens
- Parfum (fragrance)
- PEG compounds
- Petrolatum
- Sulfates
- Siloxanes
- Sodium Laureth
- Triclosan

Chapter Seven

When people say they prefer organic food, what they often seem to mean is they don't want their food tainted with pesticides and their meat shot full of hormones or antibiotics. Many object to the way a few companies - Monsanto is the most famous of them - control so many of the seeds we grow.

Michael Specter

Roundup, the most-widely used herbicide, is the marketing name for the chemical glyphosate. Glyphosate is listed as a probable carcinogen by the International Agency for Research on Cancer (IARC) which is the investigative arm of the World Health Organization (WHO). Bloomberg Business reports that the WHO has stated there is limited evidence that glyphosate causes Non-Hodgkin's lymphoma and lung cancer, but convincing evidence that it causes cancer in laboratory animals. (22)

Glyphosate also caused DNA and chromosomal damage in human cells, although it gave negative results in tests using bacteria. One study in community residents reported increases in blood markers of chromosomal damage after glyphosate formulations were sprayed nearby. (23)

Glyphosate is used in forestry, urban, and home applications. The average population is exposed primarily through residences near sprayed areas, in water, and in food. The levels observed have been low doses. However, it is important to remember Linda Birnbaum's presentation to the U.S. House of Representatives regarding the effect of low-dosing exposure of endocrine disruptors (see Chapter 4).

According to a toxicology report published in 2009 by the University of Caen in France, up to 400 ppm of glyphosate are sprayed on some animal feed. They conducted an experiment in which they exposed human liver cells to four different formulations of glyphosate, checking for cytotoxicity as well as adaptations of androgen and estrogen activity. Endocrine disruption was observed at 0.5 ppm, cytotoxic effects started at 10 ppm and DNA damage began at 5 ppm. Real cell impact of glyphosate-based herbicide residues in food, feed or in the environment has to be considered, and their classifications as carcinogens/mutagens needs to be discussed. (24) (25)

A spokesman for Monsanto, the company that produces Roundup, said: "All labeled uses of glyphosate are safe for human health," but they have gone as far as requesting a retraction of the IARC report. Critics of the company say that Monsanto has consistently covered up its toxic effects. (26)

Another peer-reviewed article, published on March 24, 2015 ties this product to antibiotic resistance. Increasingly common chemicals, which include glyphosate, used in agriculture, domestic gardens, and public places can induce a multiple-antibiotic resistance in pathogens such as *E Coli* and *Salmonella*. (26)

In order to protect our crops from the hazardous chemical in this product, Monsanto has created crops that are resistant to pesticides. They had to be genetically modified (GM) in order for this to be accomplished. An additional concern with genetically modified organisms (GMO foods) is that their seeds are able to be patented and therefore the manufacturer is technically able to control the world's food population as the demand for crops resistant to pests increases.

GM foods have the potential to affect human health, including the digestive system of the human body. GM foods have been genetically modified to resist insects and other pests, but leave residue behind that affect the ecosystem as well as humans. Monsanto leads the world in GMOs and has infiltrated its way into various high-level positions in the United States government. The former vice president of public policy, and chief lobbyist for Monsanto, was also the FDA senior advisor. He oversaw the creation of the GMO policy. According to Jeffrey Smith, a leading spokesperson on the dangers of GMO foods,

"If GMOs are indeed responsible for massive sickness and death, then the individual who oversaw the FDA policy that facilitated their introduction holds a uniquely infamous role in human history. He had been Monsanto's attorney before becoming policy chief at the FDA. Soon after, he became their vice president and chief lobbyist." (27)

According to Smith, he oversaw the policy that was responsible for the genetically engineered bovine growth hormone (rbGH) and determined that milk from injected cows did not require special labeling. He allowed this company to sue dairies that label their products "rbGH free". (28) The former FDA advisor denies his involvement, stating nothing could be further from the truth. (57)

The majority of GM crops such as soybeans, corn, canola, and sunflower seeds are now coated with neonicotinoid pesticides. Neonicotinoids are powerful neurotoxins that travel through the plants and kill insects at roots and leaves. They are also blamed for the killing of pollinators such as bees and butterflies. Neonicotinoids were found in every Midwestern stream tested. (58)

Monsanto is leading the world into a new age of potentially hazardous genetic modification of seeds. Not only have they patented their own GMO seeds, but also a huge number of crop seeds, patenting living organisms without a vote of the people or Congress. According to Dr. Joseph Mercola, they do not allow farmers to save their seeds to replant the following year and they aggressively seek out and sue farmers they suspect of doing so. (59) (60)

Chapter Eight

I treat myself pretty good. I take lots of vacations. I eat well. I take supplements. I do mercury detox. I get plenty of sleep. I drink plenty of water, and I stay away from drama and stress.
Reba McEntire

The presence of heavy metals is plentiful in the earth's crust, therefore will be present in some foods. We humans absorb these metals in trace amounts; and some metals such as zinc, copper, and selenium, are critical to maintaining the body's metabolism. At high concentrations, however, they can be dangerous to our health and can cause poisoning, mental illness, central nervous system damage and organ failure. Long term exposure may lead to cancer and death.

Arsenic, cadmium, mercury, and inorganic tin account for a majority of the cases in heavy metal poisoning. Recently, there has been a growing concern about arsenic in apple juice. We need to understand that there are organic and inorganic metals. Organic arsenic present in fruit juices has been able to pass through the body quickly and not linger in our organs. Inorganic arsenic, which comes from herbicides and pesticides, is toxic.

You may recall, from Chapter 2, my experience with mercury. The presence of inorganic tin alerted my doctor to the fact that it was coming from my fillings as opposed to fish, but I still needed to limit eating tuna to a few times per month.

Fish containing the highest amount of mercury that should be eaten sparingly throughout the year are Mackerel (King), Marlin, Orange Roughy, Shark, Swordfish, Tilefish, Tuna (Bigeye, Ahi). Pregnant women should avoid this list entirely.

The following fish should be eaten 3x per month or less: Bluefish, Grouper Mackerel (Spanish, Gulf), Sea Bass (Chilean), Tuna (Canned Albacore), and Tuna (Yellowfin).

Eat six servings or less per month of Bass (Striped, Black), Carp, Cod (Alaskan), Croaker (White Pacific), Halibut (Atlantic), Halibut (Pacific), Jacksmelt, (Silverside), Lobster, Mahi Mahi, Monkfish, Perch (Freshwater), Sablefish, Skate, Snapper, Tuna (Canned chunk light), Tuna (Skipjack), Weakfish (Sea Trout)

Fish that contain the least amount of mercury and can be enjoyed regularly are Anchovies, Butterfish, Catfish, Clam, Crab (Domestic), Crawfish/Crayfish, Croaker (Atlantic), Flounder, Haddock, (Atlantic, Hake, Herring, Mackerel (N. Atlantic, Chub), Mullet, Oyster, Perch (Ocean), Plaice, Pollock, Salmon, (Canned), Salmon (Fresh), Sardine, Scallop, Shad (American), Shrimp, Sole (Pacific), Squid, (Calamari), Tilapia, Trout (Freshwater), Whitefish, Whiting. (32)

Let's go back for a moment to our drinking water. We need the minerals from it, but not the heavy metals or the endocrine disruptors. It is much better and safer to install a good water filtration system to reduce the harmful toxins that come through your tap. Municipalities filter bacteria, but have not been very effective in filtering chemicals that disrupt our endocrine system.

Consider the current events in Flint, Michigan. In 2014, the state decided that the best use of its money would be to switch the drinking water supply from Lake Huron to the Flint River, notorious for its filth. It was supposed to be a temporary fix while a new state-run supply line was put in place. But soon after the switch, residents noted the smell was off, the taste was bad and the color was brown. The brown was not sewage. It was iron. What was not seen was far worse. Many of the service lines to the homes in Flint are made of lead and because the water was not properly treated, the lead leached into the drinking supply. A 2011 study found that it needed to be treated with an anti-corrosive agent for it to be considered as a safe source for drinking water, but it was overlooked. (46)

In Sebring, Ohio, schools were shut down in January 2016 after tests revealed lead levels at 21 parts per billion (ppb) in some homes, as compared to 27 ppb in Flint. Federal regulations are 15 ppb. (47)

The EPA says between 10% to 20% of lead exposure comes from contaminated drinking water. Babies are the most susceptible, getting 40%-60% of their exposure to lead from contaminated water mixed with formulas. Lead is not filtered out of the body. It "bio-accumulates" meaning it builds up in the body and becomes toxic.

How do you know if your water contains lead? You

can start by calling your municipal water supplier and ask for a copy of their Consumer Confidence Report, which lists levels of contaminants found during tests. Some public water suppliers put annual reports online and are accessible by typing in your zip code on the EPA's website at epa.gov.ccr. All lead levels need to fall below 15 ppb. If you discover the lead reading at higher than acceptable readings, you should contact your water supplier and ask if the service pipe at your street, or the header pipe, contains lead.

If the answer is yes, before using any water in your home, run all water faucets on cold for 5 minutes as lead levels increase with the heated water coming out of the pipes. Boiling water may remove some contaminants but it raises lead levels.

If the answer is no, it is still possible to have lead in your water because it is odorless and tasteless. Ask your local supplier to come out and test the water. Some suppliers will do it for free. You can also purchase a home test kit. If you choose to home test, follow directions for first-draw water. Water that has been left to sit the night will have the highest accumulation of toxins if there is any. You will then send the results to a lab specified on the EPA's website.

Some water filters do not filter lead. You will need to filter your water through filtering systems, reverse osmosis or distillation. Pitcher-type filters will filter some contaminants but not lead. (48)

The use of fluoride is hotly debated, and I will not get into that in this book. However, even the best of water filtration systems may not be great at filtering fluoride that is added to tap water. We use a PUR water filter system. It is affordable but it may not filter everything out. We do have our eye on a Berkey water filtration system, which is an upgrade from our PUR. Water distillation is an option for some, but not for all. It takes 5 hours to distill one gallon of water. We used to distill our water, but it made our small house very hot as it put out a lot of heat and used a good deal of electricity. Friends of ours distilled their water in an outdoor alcove.

So, what is the best drinking water? First, we need to understand the difference between filtered, purified, and distilled.

Distilled water is water created through the process of distillation. It is steamed and then separated from its contaminants and recaptured. But many of these contaminants have very high melting points, and even higher boiling points than the boiling point of water at 212 degrees F. So as the pure water is turned into steam, the junk left behind are the contaminants. But many of these are VOC's like pesticides and herbicides and are produced in the steam with the water as the water is recaptured. It is best to have an additional method of purification.

Deionized water is water that has had all the ions removed. The only thing this is beneficial for is chemistry experiments since ions may interfere with other chemicals.

Purified water is water that has had impurities reduced to very low levels. Purified water cannot contain any solids over 10 parts per million (ppm). It is cleansed and filtered through several purification processes, such as reverse osmosis, distillation or deionization. The result is water that has a higher purity than even spring water. Reverse osmosis is another purification process and uses less energy and heat than distillation.

Most bottled water is either "purified" or "drinking water." It comes from a municipal source, such as Pepsi's Aquafina or Coke's Dasani. If your bottled water isn't at least purified, you have tap water from a random municipal source. You are paying high prices for tap water that may not have that additional filtration. (29)

In addition, the plastic from the bottles contribute to the BPA that is found in our water supply. BPA stands for bisphenol A and is an industrial chemical used to make plastics and resins. Recently, many health food stores have been carrying BPA free bottles. It is much safer and more cost effective to purchase one of these and fill it with your purified, filtered tap water.

Chapter Nine

The best advice is to avoid foods with health claims on the label, or better yet, avoid foods with labels in the first place.
Mark Hyman

Product labels are important to understand. Not everything that is labeled "natural" is safer. For example, when the label reads "natural flavoring," what comes to your mind? Safe? Better? Non-toxic? Absorbable? The FDA is currently calling for comments on the meaning of this word. You may be surprised to learn that heavy metals are naturally occurring, therefore natural, and castoreum is as well.

Castoreum, according to Winter, is "a creamy, orange-brown substance with a strong, penetrating odor or bitter taste that consists of the dried perineal glands of the beaver and their secretion. The glands and secretions are taken from the area between the vulva and the anus in the female beaver and from the scrotum and the anus in the male beaver." (42) You would not find castoreum on food labels, however. It is marketed under "natural flavors" and that would not be a lie. It might be found as a substitute in vanilla products such as non-dairy creamer or ice cream. It might also be found in raspberry flavored drinks. (41) Foods labeled as "all-natural" may be injected with sodium to enhance flavor, or have high volume of high-fructose corn syrup.

"Multigrain" is another misleading food label. When you see this word you may think it is healthy. It is a marketing word that usually means that more than one grain has been used in the making of the product, usually refined, stripped of nutrients and enhanced with vitamins and minerals. It is stripped in order to allow for better digestion, but synthetic vitamins and minerals are added back, and quite often these enrichments are not readily absorbed by the body.

"No sugar added" sounds like it is low in sugar but in fact, sugar may be hidden in added ingredients like maltodextrin. "Sugar Free" does not mean lower in calories nor healthier. It may be full of artificial sweeteners. It often means that fat has been added to enhance the flavor. Sugar alcohols such as xylitol, maltitol, sorbitol, and mannitol are added in place of sugar. These sugar alcohols do have traces of sugar but they are less than .5 grams per serving, which are not required to be listed as sugar. The calories are less, but they are added back in other ingredients. I am unable to tolerate foods, such as imitation crab meat, due to the sugar alcohol added. They often cause severe gastrointestinal upset in many people.

"Zero Trans Fat" is another misleading label. Trans-fats are bad for your heart. There may be less than .5 grams per serving of trans-fat, but if you had two servings, you would be adding 1 gram of trans-fat to your diet without realizing it.

If you think you are safe because you have eaten "fat-free" then think again. You have consumed a product that more than likely is loaded with sugar and higher calories.

"Gluten free" has been all the rage in the past few years because of excellent marketing. I eat gluten-free often, but it is because I have grown intolerant to some wheat products. Gluten contains a protein called gliadin which is found in wheat, rye, and barley, and other flours if produced in the same facility due to cross-contamination. One day, however, I noticed while strolling through my local health food store and employer for 3 years, that many products on the shelf were labeled gluten free, even though their supposed 'gluten" counterpart never actually contained gluten. Because of the gluten free label, manufacturers can hike the price knowing that they will get it. People who are looking to eat healthier usually go gluten free. I am not a chemist or doctor, so my sharing this opinion is as one with an intolerance to *high amounts* of gluten: Unless you have been diagnosed with Celiac Disease, or you have sensitivities to gluten, "gluten-free" is not healthier, tastier, nor cheaper.

"Cholesterol-free" does not mean no cholesterol at all. Cholesterol-free products must contain less than 2 mg of cholesterol per serving and low cholesterol products must contain less than 20 mg per serving. If you have several helpings you had cholesterol in your diet. In addition, the liver produces cholesterol, so only animal products contain it. If you find plant-based products such as oils that are labeled "cholesterol-free" it is meaningless. Current thinking disputes whether cholesterol from foods is a problem at all, but the American Heart Association recommends no more than 300 mg of cholesterol from foods daily.

"Natural or All-Natural" meats mean that the meat is minimally processed.

"Naturally-raised" should be followed by a specific statement such as "without growth hormones or antibiotics."

"Grass-fed" is a term that claims the animals are fed solely on a diet of grass or hay and have continuous outdoor access. Cattle are natural ruminants that eat grass, so they are healthier and leaner this way. Grain fed cattle often become sickened and need antibiotics or growth hormones. Grass-fed beef has been shown to have higher amounts of healthy omega-3 fatty acids. The label should also include a certified organic label to verify it was not eating grass exposed to or treated with synthetic pesticides and fertilizers.

One term that is reliable and consistently applied is "organic," however, with specifications. Organic produce has higher vitamin and mineral content because the soil has been worked and nourished to include minerals that may have been depleted from it due to overuse or poor quality. They are also free of herbicides and pesticides. It is important to understand the various organic labels. (49)

"100% organic" means the food is completely organic and may display the USDA Organic Seal or "Certified Organic" labeling.

"Organic" means that the item must have an ingredients list; the contents should be 95% or more *certified organic*, meaning free of synthetic additives like pesticides, chemical fertilizers, and dyes; and they must not be processed using industrial solvents, irradiation, or genetic engineering, according to the USDA. The remaining 5% may only be foods processed with additives on an approved list. Water, for example, is not organic. Minerals are not organic. (30)

"Made with organic ingredients" means the item must contain 70% or more organic ingredients; the USDA seal cannot be used anywhere on the package; and the remaining 30% of the ingredients may not be foods processed with additives on a special exclusion list. Products that have less than 70% organic ingredients will be unable to carry the USDA organic seal.

PLU codes are four or five-digit numbers that identify different types of produce. For example, #4011 is the code for a standard yellow banana. The number 9 prefix added to a PLU signifies that an item is organic. For example, #94011 is the code for an organic yellow banana. A number 8 prefix added to a PLU signifies that an item is genetically engineered (GE). For example, #84011 is the code for a genetically engineered yellow banana. PLU codes and their organic prefixes are in wide use, but GE codes are rare at best.

Choosing organic can be a little more expensive than conventional foods. The cost of organic labeling and testing is shared by farmer and consumer, for starters. The organic farmer does not receive government subsidies and incentives as do other farmers, therefore the cost to the organic farmer to bring the consumer a product that is grown in mineral-rich soil and free of pesticides is considerably higher.

Recently, I had a conversation with my niece, Miranda, about the economics of eating healthy. She asked how we can afford to purchase good food when a salad at McDonald's is about $7 but a hamburger is $1. Her question was not "Why is a salad $7 and a hamburger $1?" but "How can we afford to eat healthy when the prices of healthy foods are priced in such ways to keep us from choosing healthier options?"

That's a very good question and one almost all of us have asked. It is much cheaper if you look at dollar value alone. But when you are choosing a healthier lifestyle, you must take in your entire income and outgo.

When we eat real, organic, whole foods, our cells are being nourished. We have believed the lie in America (and around much of the world), that we are hungry when our stomach is empty or about to be empty. Real hunger is when our cells are deprived of nutrition.

Whole food satisfies, and our cells are nourished. Chemically-processed, pesticide laden foods do not satisfy our cells, but rather, our taste buds and our bellies. So, we eat a lot because we think we are hungry when we feel an emptiness in our bellies, but real starvation is when our cells have received no nutrition. Our need for more is due in part to the idea that we have to feed our belly in order to escape hunger, and this contributes to the high grocery bill each week. But once we have gotten into the habit of eating healthy, some people find their overall food bill drops each week because they are able to eat less. Others who eat organically may attest to a lower overall doctor bill, and overall prescription medication bill. That is because our cells have received nutrition and much sickness is related to poor nutrition. We can be satisfied. We can say "no thanks" to seconds and in between meal junk foods. That hunger feeling that we think is hunger is not always hunger, but may often be related to the emotional ties we have to food.

As you prepare to make healthier choices, at first, it may overwhelm your pocketbook. You could start a garden. If you don't have enough land space for a garden, a container garden is wonderful on a porch or balcony; or if there is a co-op in your community, you might look into that. Some community gardens will allow you to grow a plot, or even a nearby farm may lend you land. I have friends who volunteer their time with Sustainable Agriculture Entrepreneurs (SAGE), where they learn to create ethical and sustainable foods, and deal with challenges of weeds, pests and erosion without compromising the land or their health.

I use organic "pesticides" such as Dr. Bronner's Castile Soap and water, diluted ¼ cup of soap to 1 quart of water. The upside is there are no harmful chemicals and pests hate the soap. The downside is it will need to be resprayed after a rain but it is so worth it.

While you are making the adjustment to a healthier lifestyle, and arranging your budget, you should familiarize yourself with foods from two lists called the Dirty Dozen and the Clean Fifteen, put together by the Environmental Working Group (EWG). Foods on the Dirty Dozen list should always be organic because pesticide residues seep into the produce, making it virtually impossible to remove.

According to the EWG, the Dirty Dozen for 2015 are apples, peaches, nectarines, strawberries, grapes, celery, spinach, sweet bell peppers, cucumbers, cherry tomatoes, imported snap peas and potatoes.

Each of these foods tested positive for a number of different pesticide residues and showed higher concentrations of pesticides than other produce items.

Key findings:

- 99 percent of apple samples, 98 percent of peaches, and 97 percent of nectarines tested positive for at least one pesticide residue.
- The average potato had more pesticides by weight than any other produce.
- A single grape sample and a sweet bell pepper sample contained 15 pesticides.
- Single samples of cherry tomatoes, nectarines, peaches, imported snap peas and strawberries showed 13 different pesticides apiece.

Although leafy greens such as kale and collards are not on the list, the EWG has found, for the third year in a row, trace amounts of two types of highly hazardous insecticides that are toxic to the nervous system of humans. EWG recommends buying these organically as well.

The Clean Fifteen list of produce least likely to hold pesticide residues consists of avocados, sweet corn, pineapples, cabbage, frozen sweet peas, onions, asparagus, mangoes, papayas, kiwis, eggplant, grapefruit, cantaloupe, cauliflower and sweet potatoes. Relatively few pesticides were detected on these foods, and tests found low total concentrations of pesticides on them.

Key findings:

- Avocados were the cleanest: only 1 percent of avocado samples showed any detectable pesticides.

- Some 89 percent of pineapples, 82 percent of kiwi, 80 percent of papayas, 88 percent of mango and 61 percent of cantaloupe had no residues.

- No single fruit sample from the Clean 15 tested positive for more than 4 types of pesticides.

- Multiple pesticide residues are extremely rare on Clean 15 vegetables. Only 5.5 percent of Clean 15 samples had two or more pesticides. (31)

Since U.S. law does not require labeling of genetically engineered produce, EWG advises people who want to avoid GE crops to purchase organically-grown foods or items bearing the "Non-GMO Project Verified" label.

Based upon these lists, I also suggest berries of any kind be purchased organically.

Chapter Ten

I did research when I was pregnant with my first daughter and was horrified by the chemicals in products, even those meant for babies. I would have to go to 50 different places just to get my house and my kid clean.

Jessica Alba

I had been asked, "If you could choose just one household cleaning product to keep on hand, what would that be?" My answer would be, "hydrogen peroxide." I admit, I used to say it was white vinegar, but I have changed my mind (for the benefit of all those who have sat in on my classes). Hydrogen peroxide (H_2O_2) is an all-natural product that is produced by enzymes in the human body. But since H_2O_2 can be damaging to the human tissues, it is contained within specialized organelles called peroxisomes. These peroxisomes contain enzymes called catalase which will break down peroxide should it be possible to escape. It is produced to keep cells healthy. When the immune system is activated in response to bacteria, hydrogen peroxide is produced to fight infection.

As a household ingredient, hydrogen peroxide is diluted to about 3% so it isn't as caustic. However, it is still very useful as an antibacterial, antimicrobial, antifungal, and antiseptic agent. You can substitute hydrogen peroxide for chlorine bleach in routine maintenance cleaning. But, I'll bet you didn't know that hydrogen peroxide is also excellent for washing windows, mirrors, glass surfaces, stove tops, stainless steel and shower doors. It works better than vinegar. Spray it on tile after a shower to keep it from getting mildew. Spray your shower head and leave it. No need to rinse. It works great as a whitening agent on grout.

Hydrogen peroxide must be left in a dark container, as the light will render it ineffective. I had purchased a small bottle with a sprayer in Dollar General, but you can purchase a bottle and put your own sprayer on. I love to add a few drops of essential oils, such as pine *(Pinus sylvestris)* or lemon (*Citrus limon*).

I do opt for vinegar on floors. It doesn't matter if it is white vinegar or cider vinegar. However white vinegar has a less potent smell. To mask some of the vinegar smell, I like to add a few drops of essential oil (any fragrance) but be sure to test a small patch on your floor to be sure the essential oils do not harm the finish. Vinegar is also considered an antibacterial, antiviral, antimicrobial.

I love Dr. Bronner's Castile Soap as a surfactant. A surfactant lowers the water's surface tension which means it helps it to spread out and penetrate more easily. I will often mix about 2 – 4 ounces of water and 1 tablespoon of castile soap when cleaning countertops because it helps to remove stuck on food and grease. I also add essential oils to this mix as well; about 5 drops per ounce of water.

Baking soda (sodium bicarbonate) is another product produced in the human body. It is used to help keep the body out of acidic state. Without sufficient bicarbonates, the pancreas is slowly destroyed. The link between metabolic acidosis and diabetes is sodium bicarbonates. Even 1 teaspoon in a glass of water helps reduce stomach upset and gas. In housecleaning, baking soda is useful as a soft scrub – just add a little water sufficient to make a paste and scrub away. Be careful to rinse well as it does leave a film behind. It is great in conjunction with vinegar as a drain unclogger. Pour baking soda first, then vinegar, down the drain and let it sit for about 30 minutes.

As a carpet deodorizer I mix up baking soda and essential oil. Shake well. As a carpet stain remover, baking soda on the stained area for about 5 minutes should remove minor stains. But for tougher stains, spray vinegar on top of the baking soda and check every five minutes. Vacuum when dry.

My suggestion is to start with these basics. You may find that you want to purchase an all-natural product for certain tasks; but if you start with these, you might find these products to be all you need. Not only are they cost-effective, but they are useful for personal care as well.

Recipe – Carpet Deodorizer

- 1 c aluminum free baking soda

- 1 tsp lavender oil *Lavandula angustifolia* (or fragrance of your choice)

Shake well so that essential oil is evenly distributed. I use an empty grated cheese dispenser. Sprinkle throughout carpet. Vacuum after 5 minutes.

Recipe- Floor Cleaner

- 2 parts filtered or distilled water

- 1 part white vinegar

- Optional – 10 drops essential oil of your choice per ounce of liquid (test on a small section of floor)

Recipe- All-purpose spray

- Spray bottle of hydrogen peroxide

- Optional - 10 drops essential oil per ounce of liquid

- Optional – 1 tsp. Dr. Bronner's Castile Soap per 4 ounces liquid

*for glass and mirrors, do not add essential oil or soap.

Chapter Eleven

Drink warm water with lemon first thing in the morning. It's a good way to detox and alkalize your body.

Valentina Zelyaeva

In 1904, a Russian naturopathic physician named Ilya Metchnikoff discovered that the body would recycle whatever toxin it could not purge via the elimination pathways. These pathways are the lungs, liver, kidneys, skin, colon, lymph and blood. Each of these pathways works with the others to break down and eliminate toxins from the body. If one of the pathways is compromised in any way, it places greater burden on the other pathways. Constipation is an example of the colon not functioning to its fullest capacity. Edema in the tissues is an example of the kidneys, lymph and skin not functioning to their fullest capacity. Bloating, belching, and flatulence (gas) are the result of the liver not functioning well. Poor circulation is an example of the blood pathway not functioning. The key to good health is to know these seven pathways and do whatever it takes to keep them functioning optimally.

The Liver

The function of the liver is to break down everything that enters the body and redistribute it to other organs or pathways. Toxins will be distributed to the kidneys or colon; but when it gets overloaded, it tries to utilize every other elimination system until they become full. The liver chemically converts destructive toxins into less harmful substances that the colon and kidneys can eliminate. When toxins fail to be eliminated due to overburdening of the pathways, they are then sent to the fat cells to be stored. (33)

Helpful foods and herbs for liver support are milk thistle (*silybum marianum*), artichoke leaf (*Cynara scolymus*), dandelion root (*Taraxacum oficinales*), ashwagandha (*Withania somnifera*) and garlic (*Allium sativum*). Dandelion root is widely available in our backyards (but only collect what is about 100 feet away from roads to protect from possible pesticide contamination from neighboring yards or spray trucks). The greens are bitter and can be added to salads, or steamed and added with other greens. As a tea, dandelion root has a nutty flavor.

Recipe – Dandelion Root Tea (*Taraxacum officinale*)

Gather the whole plant, from the root and wash well. Choose dandelions about 100 feet away from the road or from your neighbor's lawn. The root is long so it may take a little patience digging it up.

Separate the root from the leaves and chop the root coarsely. Bring 1 quart of water to a boil in a saucepan and add 2 teaspoons of the root. Cover and lower the heat to simmer for about 1 minute.

Remove from heat and let steep for about 40 minutes. You may add the leaves and flowers about 5-7 minutes before you are ready to strain it.

Strain by placing a strainer over your teacup and pour. Add a little honey as desired.

Drinking a few cups daily will help cleanse your liver and support its function. Many of these other herbs are available as teas that you can sip on for added cleansing benefits. Juicing green vegetables with lemon and ginger (*Zingibar officinale*) is a great detoxifying tonic.

Turmeric (*Curcuma longa*) helps protect the liver from inflammation and boosts liver cell regeneration. Research has also shown that artichoke leaf supports detoxification by stimulating bile while protecting liver cells from free radicals (highly reactive compounds that can cause damage to cells).

Beets, carrots, cruciferous and leafy vegetables, olive oil, avocados, green tea, turmeric, and cabbage are excellent to add to a juice. Lemons, limes and apples are good too, but keep sweeter fruit to a minimum if sugar is a problem for you. The temptation to make juices very sweet is often there, but too much sugar is hard on the liver, even fruit sugar. Fructose (fruit sugar) can be damaging to the body because it lacks the fiber from the fruit and will cause a quick release of insulin in response to the quickly-absorbing sugar into the bloodstream. I like using a NutriBullet because the fiber remains and therefore the sugar from any fruit is slowly absorbed, thus insulin is released more slowly into the body. If you choose to juice with a juicer that removes the fiber, stick with 2 ounces daily, preferably in the morning, using one or two fruits and add more greens. I like to make "juice cubes." I add them to the water that I drink throughout the day.

Greatly reduce, or avoid if possible, the consumption of Tylenol, Ibuprofen, or Advil, and caffeine (on a regular basis), sugar, grains, processed foods, and alcohol as these can damage the liver. Harvard Medical School has an eye-opening list of the top twelve pain relievers and their effects on the body on their website. (50)

Turmeric and ginger, as a food, a tea or in supplement form, are great pain alternative pain relievers.

Recipe- Turmeric Rice (*adapted from Food.com*) (52)

- 2 tsp Coconut Oil
- ½ c diced Onions
- 1 c "non-enriched" Rice such as brown rice
- ¼ tsp powdered Turmeric or 1 tsp fresh Turmeric (*Curcuma longa*)
- ¼ tsp ground Cumin (*Cuminum cyminum*)
- 2 Garlic Cloves, minced
- 2 ½ c Chicken stock or water
- Seasonings

Heat saucepan and add coconut oil. When oil has melted, add onions until translucent. Add rice, turmeric, cumin and garlic. Sauté about 2 minutes and add the stock. Bring to a boil and then turn to low heat. Cover. Cook for 45 minutes. Remove from heat and leave lid on for 5 minutes. Fluff.

The Skin

Sweating is the body's way of cooling down once it is heated up. But sweating has another function. The skin disposes of more waste by sweating, because of its large surface area, than the kidneys and colon combined. Sweating is used therapeutically to help lower levels of systemic mold, mycotoxins, and heavy metals like mercury. It's also an effective exit route for environmental toxins like BPA, phthalates and xenoestrogens. (34) (35)

To keep the skin healthy, try exfoliating by dry skin brushing, (You can easily look on YouTube for a demonstration of effective dry skin brushing) as well as moisturize and tone. For oily skin, use alcohol free hydrating toner or apple cider vinegar. For drier skin, coconut oil is gentle on the face, while almond, apricot and grapeseed are good for the body. Rosewater is an excellent toner.

Consider dandelion root tea as a facial wash since acne is often related to liver congestion.

Recipe – Facial Mask
- ¼ c organic ground coffee.
- Egg white from one egg
- Apply mask to face, gently massaging in a circular motion until it is spread evenly on the face.
- Wait until it dries, about 10 minutes.
- Place a warm cloth on your face for a few moments to loosen it up and rinse clean.

Do care for cuts, burns and scrapes promptly. Calendula cream, lavender oil, colloidal silver, and Aloe Vera are good to have in your natural first aid cabinet. Do not use calendula on an open wound. It is such a powerful skin healer it may heal the skin before any infection underneath has a chance to heal.

Use arrowroot powder, baking soda or coconut oil with essential oil to absorb odor and sweat at the armpit and groin areas in place of anti-perspirants or talcum powder. (36)

Avoid the use of mineral oil or Petroleum Jelly. These are byproducts of crude oil used in the manufacturing of petrol gasoline (where we get the name petrolatum or petroleum jelly from). Petroleum is used in a number of agricultural products, one being in the production of ammonia. It is used in plastic-making, tires, pharmaceuticals, dyes, detergents, vitamin capsules, denture adhesives, deodorants, lipstick, and crayons. Petroleum and petroleum-based products clog the skin, rendering it impossible for toxins to be released. (53)

Coconut oil is a great staple because it can be used to condition your hair, hydrate your skin and used in place of butter. (Not that butter is bad, I love butter, but I can eat too much). You will want to choose unrefined, expeller-pressed, extra virgin coconut oil for maximum nutritional benefits. You can find food grade coconut oil in the oils section of your supermarket. No need to also buy in the health and beauty aisle. It's more expensive there anyway.

Some helpful foods for the skin belong to the yellow,

orange, and purple food groups. Spicy foods or hot soups also open the pores and allow the sweat to happen. Helpful herbs such as green tea, turmeric, hot peppers, ginger, and mustard are delicious and skin supporting herbs to add to the daily diet.

Recipe – Curried Carrot Soup

- 2 tbsp. Butter (choose organic butter or grass fed)
- 1 c chopped Onion
- 1 tsp Curry Powder or Turmeric (*Curcuma longa*)
- 1 tsp ground Cumin (*Cuminum cyminum*)
- 1 tbsp. minced Garlic (*Allium sativum*)
- 3 ½ c Chicken Stock
- 2 lbs. Carrots, peeled and cut into small chunks
- 1 tbsp. fresh-squeezed Lemon Juice
- 2 tbsp. Cilantro (*Coriandrum sativum*) or Parsley (*Petroselinum crispum*) for garnish

Heat butter in a large saucepan or Dutch oven, over medium heat. Add onion, turmeric, cumin and garlic. Salt and pepper to taste. Cook until onion is soft, about 5 minutes. Add broth, carrots and 3 cups of water then bring to a boil. Reduce heat and simmer until carrots are tender, about 20 minutes.

In a blender, (or hand held mixer) puree the soup in batches until smooth. Add more or less water to thin or thicken. Stir in lemon juice.

The Blood

Healthy blood circulation is crucial to removing toxins from the body. That is because the blood transports toxins to other organs for proper elimination. Massage is beneficial for stimulating blood circulation as well as lymph flow.

Red clover (*Trifolium pretense*), a perennial herb native to Europe, Central Asia and northern Africa, has been used traditionally as a blood purifier with beneficial results.

Some foods that are good for blood purification are those high in vitamin c and omega 3's, such as lemons, salmon, avocados, olive oil, almonds, lentils, tomatoes, and leafy greens.

Herbs such as hawthorn berry (*Crataegus monynga*), red clover (*Trifolium pretense*) alfalfa (*Medicago sativa*), hibiscus (*Rosa sinensis*), kelp, green tea (those on blood thinning medications need to consult physician before taking) are very good in a tea.

Recipe – Blood Tonic (a Darlene Rose original blend)

- 1 part Hibiscus (*Rosa sinensis*)
- 1 part Red Rooibos (*Aspalathus linearis*)
- 1 part Passionflower (*Passiflora foetida*)
- ¼ part Organic Citrus Peel (*Citrus limonum*)
- ¼ part Oatstraw (*Avena sativum*)
- ¼ part Anise seed (*Pimpinella anisum*)
- 1/8 part true Ceylon cinnamon (*Cinnamomum verum*)

Blend well. Pour 1 ounce boiling water over 1 tablespoon dried herbs. Steep for 15 minutes. Drink. Daily consumption may help reduce blood pressure as well.

Avoid foods that have trans-fats. Refined carbohydrates elevate blood pressure, cholesterol, and insulin. Insulin further increases triglycerides (blood fat), cholesterol and blood pressure. The blood becomes slow and sticky and the situation is ripe for clotting.

Recipe – Zucchini, Fennel and White Bean Pasta (high in iron) (adapted from Eatingwell.com) (51)

- 1 tbsp. Fennel seed (*Foeniculum vulgarae*)
- 2 medium Zucchini
- 3 tbsp. extra virgin cold-pressed Olive Oil
- ¼ tsp fine Sea Salt or Himalayan salt
- 8 ounces whole wheat or gluten free Pasta (short)
- 2 cloves Garlic, minced or finely chopped
- 1 c cooked cannellini beans
- 2 plum tomatoes
- ¾ c hard cheese such as Romano or goat cheese
- Freshly ground pepper and salt to taste

Preheat oven to 400°F.

Quarter zucchini lengthwise. Toss the fennel and zucchini with 1 tablespoon oil and salt. Arrange in a single layer on a large baking sheet. Roast, turning once, until soft and beginning to brown, about 20 minutes.

Meanwhile, bring a large pot of water to a boil. Add pasta; cook until just tender, 8 to 10 minutes or according to package directions.

Heat the remaining 2 tablespoons oil in a large skillet over medium heat. Add garlic and cook, stirring, for 30 seconds. Remove from the heat.

When the vegetables are cool enough to handle, coarsely chop. Add the vegetables, beans and ½ cup bean-cooking liquid (or other liquid) to the pan with the garlic and place over medium-low heat. Drain the pasta and immediately add it to the pan.

Toss thoroughly and add tomatoes; toss until just warm. Remove from the heat and stir in cheese. Season with salt and pepper to taste.

Where the salt goes, the water flows. Salt, potassium, and water are necessary for proper blood pressure and heart function. Many diets that are supportive for the heart restrict salt in order to reduce the water that collects in the tissues and can cause heart disease. The body, however, needs a proper balance of salt, potassium and water in order to function. When you drink too much water, salt is diluted, and tissues start to swell up. If you drink a lot of water to help your kidneys, add a teaspoon or two of fresh lemon juice (not bottled lemon juice) so as not to cause an unhealthy imbalance of electrolytes. Himalayan salt has 84 minerals and is properly balanced. It also helps balance the body's PH levels, while regular salt promotes acidity.

Take hot showers or baths, not scalding. It increases oxygen in the tissues and promotes circulation.

The Lymphatic System

The lymphatic system needs outside stimulation. It transports lymph, a clear, colorless fluid that contains white blood cells used to fight infection. It is comprised of the lymph vessels, lymph nodes and lymph. The tonsils, adenoids, spleen, thymus and about six to seven hundred lymph nodes are all part of this network that is responsible for ridding the body of toxins.

The lymphatic system transports wastes and toxins from cells and the circulatory system to each of the organs involved in the elimination of toxins from the body. This system of vessels carries immune cells in a network that follows the body's bloodstream. While your circulatory system, which transports red blood cells, circulates on its own, lymph travels upward toward the neck and empties into the venous blood stream which is near your clavicles. Infected lymph nodes will cause glands to be swollen, and the lymph becomes stagnant. Lymph needs stimulation because it carries toxins and these toxins can slow drainage process. You can support the flow of lymph by dry-brushing daily or by using a rebounder, trampoline, doing aerobics or cardio exercise, and getting massages.

Green tea is an excellent antioxidant that helps the lymphatic system further release toxins. Spirulina, wheatgrass (*Elymus scaber*) and chlorophyll have also been shown to help the function of immune cells found in lymph.

The Lungs

The lungs purge toxins from the body each time you

exhale. Deep breathing increases the flow of lymph, and helps to eliminate toxins. Practice deep breathing exercises at least 10 minutes per day, some form or cardio, rebounding, or aerobic exercise.

To properly deep breathe, place one hand on the chest and the other on the belly. Take a deep breath in through the nose, to a count of 6, then exhale through the nose also to a count of 8. Exhaling through the nose adds a natural resistance to the breath. By holding one hand on your belly and the other on your chest, you are ensuring the diaphragm (not the chest) inflates with enough air to create a stretch in the lungs. The goal is six to 10 deep, slow breaths per minute for 10 minutes each day to experience immediate reductions to heart rate and blood pressure. Keep at it for six to eight weeks, and those benefits might stick around even longer.

Stop Smoking Now! It's not too late – EVER! There are over 4000 carcinogenic chemicals in tobacco smoke, including 69 known carcinogenic compounds, according to the American Lung Association. Here are some other chemicals found in tobacco smoke:

- Acetone – found in nail polish remover

- Acetic Acid – an ingredient in hair dye

- Ammonia – a common household cleaner

- Arsenic – used in rat poison

- Benzene – found in rubber cement

- Butane – used in lighter fluid

- Cadmium – active component in battery acid

- Carbon Monoxide – released in car exhaust fumes

- Formaldehyde – embalming fluid

- Hexamine – found in barbecue lighter fluid

- Lead – used in batteries

- Naphthalene – an ingredient in moth balls

- Methanol – a main component in rocket fuel

- Nicotine – used as insecticide

- Tar – material for paving roads

- Toluene - used to manufacture paint (37)

Foods that support healthy lungs are cruciferous vegetables, citrus, and carotenoids, foods high in Omega 3's such as salmon, asparagus, beets, peaches, lentils, garlic, berries, apples, and pure fresh water. One herb that helps support the lungs is mullein (*Verbascum thapsus*).

Mullein (*Verbascum thapsus*) is used to help alleviate the irritation of mucous membranes in the respiratory tract by removing the phlegm. You may find mullein growing in your backyard. It looks like a big green rosette in its first year. In the second year it grows up to 3 feet tall from the rosette, has a hairy stem and yellow flowers. If you do not have mullein, you may find it at your local health food store.

Turmeric (*Curcuma longa*) may also lower the risk of lung inflammation. Herbs that support the lungs are green tea, lungwort (*Pulmonaria officinalis*) eucalyptus (*Eucalyptus globulus*), oregano (*Origanum vulgare*), basil (*Ocimum basilicum*), garlic (*Allium sativum*), ginger (*Zingibar officinale*), and peppermint (*Mentha piperita*).

Recipe – Mullein Tea (*Verbascum thapsus*)

- 1 ½ c boiling water
- 1-2 tsp dried Mullein *(Verbascum thapsus)* leaves and/or flowers (flowers make a sweeter tea)
- 1 tsp dried Spearmint (*Mentha Canadensis*) (optional for flavor)
- 1-2 tsp Honey (optional)

Steep the mullein leaves in hot water inside a tea ball or strainer for 15 minutes. Add honey if you like a sweeter tea.

Recipe – Ginger Peach Smoothie

- 3 leaves fresh Basil (*Ocimum basilicum*)
- 14 medium Carrots
- ½ Lemon
- 5 medium Peaches
- ¼ inch fresh Ginger root (*Zingibar officinale*)

Add to a juicer in this order: Basil (*Ocimum basilicum*), lemon, peaches, carrots and ginger.

The Kidneys

The function of the kidneys is to remove liquid waste (toxins) from the body. We need to drink purified water on a daily basis to assist the kidneys in this function. The human body cannot go more than 3 days without water before it begins to shut down; but there is so much confusing advice on the internet about how much water is safe to drink. The old standard of drinking eight 8-ounce glasses of water doesn't, well excuse the pun, hold water any longer. For example, this does not take into account how old the person is, how much a person weighs, whether a person is male or female, or if one leads an active or sedentary life. A runner needs more water than a person who is sedentary (because they lose more water through sweat), and an adult needs more water than a child. A 300 lb. man would need more water than a 125 lb woman. So drink half your weight in ounces of water on an average day. For example, if you weigh 150 lbs., then half of 150 is 75; so drink 75 ounces. If you work out, you may need more than that. Don't forget to add lemon for electrolyte balance. (38)

Don't hold your water. The longer your urine is held, the more time you give bacteria opportunity to get into the urethra and even the kidneys, forming a UTI or bladder and kidney infection. So, urinate as often as you feel the urge. (39)

Supportive foods for the kidneys are red bell peppers, cabbage, cauliflower, garlic (*Allium sativum*), onions, apples, cranberries, blueberries, raspberries, cherries, red grapes, egg whites, fish, olive oil, celery, apple cider vinegar, and of course, water.

Supporting herbs are chanca piedra (*Phyllanthus niruri*) goldenrod (*Solidago virgaurea*), hydrangea root or gravel root as it is sometimes called (*Hydrangea arborescens*), horsetail (*Equisitum arvense*), celery root (*Apium graveolens*), uva ursi, sometimes called bearberry (*Arbutus uva ursi*) marshmallow root (*Althea officinalis*), dandelion root (*Taraxacum officinale*), parsley (*Apium petroselinum*), and cilantro (*Coriandrum sativum*).

Recipe – Cauliflower and Garlic Sauce (54)

- 4 c Cauliflower florets
- 2 Garlic cloves (*Allium sativum*)
- 1 tbsp. Olive Oil
- 4 tsp local, raw Honey
- 3 tbsp. apple Cider Vinegar (with the mother)
- 1 tbsp. fresh Parsley (*Apium petroselinum*)

In a large saucepan with steamer rack, steam cauliflower over boiling water 8 to 10 minutes or until crisp-tender (cover with lid while steaming). In a small saucepan, cook minced garlic in olive oil for 30 seconds, then remove pan from heat. Stir in honey, apple cider vinegar and chopped parsley. Return saucepan to heat until sauce is heated.

Transfer steamed cauliflower to a serving dish. Pour sauce over hot cauliflower and toss to coat.

The Colon

Dr. Ilya Metchnikoff, who was also considered the father of natural immunity, said "Death begins in the colon." The bowel (or colon) disposes of toxins from the digestive system and the liver, so cleansing the colon helps clear the way for other organs to function properly and help purge the body of unwanted toxins that we take in from the food we eat, the water we drink, the air we breathe, and the prescription medications we take. A colon filled with toxins can lead to constipation, weight gain, low energy, headaches, and many other illnesses and disease. Autopsies reveal the colons of 80% of people who have passed away are clogged up with waste material.

Fermented foods such as yogurt, kefir, miso, sauerkraut and kimchi help to replenish your body of beneficial bacteria. They are probiotics. Probiotics are a great start to obtaining a healthy colon. Your colon consists of trillions of bacteria. Some are beneficial. Some are not. The ideal ratio of bacteria in our bodies should be 80 % good to 20% bad. Due to our lifestyles, environment, injury, illness, processed foods and antibiotics, we are more like 80% bad and 20% good, and that is being optimistic. Having a balance in bacteria is critical to wellness. Probiotics add good bacteria, which destroy some of the bad, but it can be overwhelming to understand which probiotic is right for you. If you have a natural physician or holistic nutritionist, you may want to consult with them regarding which is right as everyone has different needs. If not, check out your local health food store for information. I take Renew Life, 30 billion strain; but I am not closed to trying others. In fact, it is suggested that you change up the brands every few months so you can add different beneficial bacteria back into your system. Good bacteria not only overpower harmful bacteria, but also help keep the body's defense mechanisms against other harmful organisms (viruses, parasites) in top shape.

A diet high in fiber helps scrub the colon clean. There are two types of fiber—soluble and insoluble. Soluble fiber is that food which is soluble in water. In other words, it expands in the body, like oats and beans. It is important to remember that this type of fiber will expand, causing you to feel full so you don't want to eat a lot. Insoluble fiber does not expand.

Insoluble Fiber

This includes whole wheat bread or cereal, wheat bran, whole grains, granola, muesli, seeds, nuts, popcorn, beans and lentils, berries, grapes and raisins, cherries, peaches, nectarines, apricots, and pears , apples, rhubarb, melon, oranges, grapefruits, lemons, limes, dates and prunes, all leafy greens, snow peas, green beans, kernel corn, bell peppers, eggplant, celery, onions, shallots, leeks, scallions and garlic, cabbage, bok choy, brussels sprouts, broccoli, cauliflower, tomatoes, cucumbers, sprouts, and fresh herbs.

Soluble Fiber

This includes rice, pasta, noodles, rice cereals, flour tortillas, white bread (not whole grain), soy, quinoa, corn meal, potatoes, carrots, yams, sweet potatoes, turnips, rutabagas, parsnips, beets, squash, pumpkins, mushrooms, chestnuts, avocados, bananas, applesauce, mangoes, and papayas.

If you have been diagnosed with Irritable Bowel Syndrome or Disorder, you will want to choose from the list of soluble fiber foods rather than the insoluble fiber list. Should you eat from the insoluble fiber list, never eat it alone or with the peels. Eat with a larger portion of soluble fiber. Trust me, it is safer. (55)

Recipe – Escarole and Bean Soup
(I love this soup. I make mine Italian style – a little of this, a little of that. I have taken the recipe below from Epicurious.com)

- 1 tbsp. Olive Oil
- 1 c chopped Onion
- 1 large carrot, cut into small dice
- 5 large Garlic (*Allium sativum*) cloves, peeled, flattened
- 3 c (packed) 1-inch pieces Escarole (about 1/2 large head)
- 4 c (or more) Chicken stock
- 3 1/4 c cooked Great Northern beans or two 15-ounce cans Cannellini (White Kidney Beans), rinsed, drained
- 1 14 1/2- to 16-ounce can diced Tomatoes, drained

(the recipe calls for canned tomatoes but fresh are preferable. BPA has been found in some food can liners, particularly canned tomatoes. For a list of canned goods with and without BPA, see inspirationgreen.com.)(56)

Heat oil in heavy large Dutch oven over medium-low heat. Add onion, carrot and garlic and sauté until onion is golden and tender, about 7 minutes. Discard garlic. Add escarole; stir 3 minutes. Add 4 cups broth, beans and tomatoes and bring to boil. Reduce heat to medium-low. Cover and simmer until escarole is tender and flavors blend, about 20 minutes. Thin with more broth, if desired. Season soup to taste with salt and pepper. Top with Romano cheese if desired.

Triphala, perhaps the most popular Ayurvedic herbal combination in India, is used to help cleanse and tone the bowel. (It is also used to cleanse the liver and blood.) It is a combination of three Ayurvedic fruits, but is taken in supplement form.

Herbs that help keep the colon clean are fennel (*Foeniculum vulgarae*), chamomile *(Matricaria recruitita)*, slippery elm (*Ulmas rubra*), milk thistle (*Silybum mariana*), dandelion (*Taraxacum officinale*), chickweed (*Stellaria media*), plantain (*Plantago major*), flaxseed (*Linum usitatissimum*), psyllium husk (Plantago psyllium), rosemary (*Rosmarinus officinalis*), and peppermint (*Mentha piperita*).

Do drink a sufficient amount of water. See **Kidneys**.

How can I escape poop when writing about the colon? I cannot. Your poop is a tell-tale sign of good or bad health. But I only learned a few years ago what to look for. First, it is optimal to poop 3-4 x per day. If you are not, you have some investigative work to do.

On the following page there is a table I used from Dr. Mercola's site. (40)

Healthy Stool	Unhealthy Stool
	Stool that is hard to pass, painful, or requires straining
Medium to light brown	
Smooth and soft, formed into one long shape and not a bunch of pieces	Hard lumps and pieces, or mushy and watery, or pasty
About one to two inches in diameter and up to 18 inches long	Narrow, pencil-like or ribbon-like stools: can indicate a bowel obstruction or tumor; and if they persist, definitely warrant a call to your physician
S-shaped, which comes from the shape of your lower intestine	Black, tarry stools or bright red stools may indicate bleeding in the GI tract; black stools can also come from certain medications, supplements or consuming black licorice
Quiet and gentle dive into the water, it should fall	White, pale or gray stools may indicate a lack of bile,

into the bowl with the slightest little "whoosh" sound – not a loud, wet cannonball splash that leaves your bottom in need of a shower	which may suggest a serious problem, so this warrants a call to your physician; antacids may produce white stool
Natural smell, not repulsive (I'm not saying it will smell good)	Yellow stools may indicate giardia infection, a gallbladder problem; if you see this, call your doctor
Uniform texture	Presence of undigested food
Sinks slowly	Floaters or splashers
	Increased mucus in stool: This can be associated with inflammatory bowel disease like Crohn's disease, or ulcerative colitis, or even colon cancer, especially if accompanied by blood or abdominal pain

Chapter Twelve

Hence the saying: If you know the enemy and you know
yourself, your victory will not stand in doubt; if you
know Heaven and you know Earth, you may make your
victory complete.
Sun Tzu

In 2011, I hired a holistic nutritionist, to help me with bloating so bad, I had to wear drawstring pants and balloon type shirts. I thought I was eating correctly. At least I was eating much better than I used to eat. I took all the really good vitamins, especially B-complex, because of my previous tremors. B-complex is very good for the nervous system and will help the body to be calm.

My nutritionist wanted me to have a blood test taken so she could determine where I was nutritionally and what, if any, deficiencies I might have. Once I sent her the results, she contacted me to ask, "Where are your B's?" She said that my blood tests revealed that I was deficient in B's. I asked for a second opinion on the test because I was taking 1000% of the RDA of B vitamins. My second opinion agreed; my tests indicated I had no B's.

Another specialist ordered a second test which indicated I was not absorbing vitamins because my gut lining, where most vitamins are absorbed, was suppressed. This is called "leaky gut." All the vitamins in the world would not do me any good because my body was not able to absorb them. Leaky gut is a symptom of the toxic effects of glyphosate. Glyphosate kills gut bacteria and allows pathogens in the body to overgrow, which many autistic children often suffer from. It interferes with the function of cytochrome P450 enzymes which detoxify toxic chemicals in the liver and if these enzymes aren't working the liver cannot break toxins down. It also interferes with the chelation of important minerals such as iron, cobalt and manganese.

Processed foods are easier. The day I made the decision to eat healthier, I didn't feel better eating broccoli and cabbage. My stomach felt tumultuous. I needed my food processed because I had poor digestion and was only able to eat what was broken down into almost mush. As I set my focus on creating a healthier gut environment, repairing my digestive system by removing what was harmful, and substituting with better choices, over time, I could eat whole foods, and even raw foods.

Changing how you do life is not easy. A bottle of ammonia spray is cheaper and more convenient. I didn't want to think about whether a product really worked. I just wanted something that said it worked; and if it was cheap and convenient, I bought it. I didn't associate my headaches with my cleaning supplies.

I didn't put much thought into cosmetics and skin care. I was young enough not to need a lot of creams and lotions. But if a lotion had a nice smell to it (if it was pleasing to my senses), it didn't matter to me what ingredients made up the smell or the lotion itself. I noticed however, that I never cracked a sweat. In fact, I could not relate to anyone who sweat at all.

We understand line upon line, precept upon precept; and as our spirit, soul and body is built up, we absorb more. We can make a decision today to change toxic patterns, but we cannot remove all chemicals nor heavy metals, go on a 40 day fast, detox, nor eat only whole foods right at the moment of our decision. Our bodies will protest the loss of what it has perceived to be delicious things. Our mind will protest the necessity of the change. That protest is a sign that the body needs to be built up, not that the lifestyle change may work for others, but not for you.

There is also grace. Now that you are aware of what these endocrine disruptors are, and how they may affect the human body, that does not mean that you will get an autoimmune disease tomorrow or ever. Pray over your food, bless it, but also understand what is in what you eat.

I have attempted to bring awareness to the fact that, over time, these endocrine disruptors slowly change the environment around you and the environment in the human body. But over time, your body will work for you when you feed it what it needs and eliminate what is harmful. The Grand Canyon was not created instantly, but by one drop of the Colorado River, every second of every minute of every day for many years.

Infirmities that remain have had a history of creeping in, secretly, slowly and over time. Healing that remains also has a history. Understanding that your body is fearfully and wonderfully made, you can decide to walk in healing, first by making the decision and then pressing in. Start slowly. Move towards a healthier, organic, endocrine disruptor-free lifestyle, one step at a time, and one day at a time. Remove one product you know you could do without and replace it with a cleaner solution. Remove one processed food from your cabinet and replace it with a healthier option. Throw away one cosmetic and replace it with an all-natural version of the same. Do one thing every day.

Your enemy is not a single chemical in a large or small dose. Your body would recognize it as foreign and fight it. Your enemy is the chronic low-dose over a period of time, because it is unseen and unsuspected.

Knowing your enemy will help keep you in the fight when it gets tough. Knowing you are not powerless will help you remain victorious in it.

References

(1) Eck, P. (1989). Mercury Toxicity. Retrieved 2014, from
http://www.arltma.com/Articles/MercuryToxDoc.htm

(2) **www.healingrooms.com

(3) Kennedy, D. (Producer). (2005, January 1). Smoking Teeth = Poison Gas [Radio series episode]. Champions Gate: International Academy of Oral Medicine and Toxicology. D.D.S.

(4) Causes of Autoimmune Disease. (n.d.). Retrieved December 23, 2015, from
http://www.evenbetterhealth.com/autoimmune-disease-causes.php

(5) VN, S. (2014, January 10). West Virginia Chemical Spill Triggers State Of Emergency, Tap Water Ban In 9 Counties Affecting 300,000 Customers; Schools, Restaurants Closed. *International Business Times*. Retrieved December 23, 2015, from http://www.ibtimes.com/west-virginia-chemical-spill-triggers-state-emergency-tap-water-ban-9-counties-1534434

(6) Official: No quick fix for West Virginia water woes - CNN.com. (2014, January 12). Retrieved December 23, 2015, from
http://www.cnn.com/2014/01/11/us/west-virginia-contaminated-water/

(7) Cocke, W. (2004, November 3). Male Fish Producing Eggs in Potomac River. Retrieved December 23, 2015, from

http://news.nationalgeographic.com/news/2004/11/
1103_041103_potomac_fish.html

(8) Male fish becoming female? (2004, November 9).
Retrieved December 23, 2015, from
http://www.nbcnews.com/id/6436617/ns/nbc_night
ly_news_with_brian_williams/t/male-fish-
becoming-female/#.Vls8sSvF_Uk

(9) Masters, R. (n.d.). Pharmaceuticals and Endocrine
Disruptors in Rivers and On Tap. Retrieved
December 23, 2015, from
http://opensiuc.lib.siu.edu/cgi/viewcontent.cgi?arti
cle=1152&context=jcwre

(10) Ward, E. (2012, July 23). Green Risks. Retrieved
December 23, 2015, from
http://greenrisks.blogspot.com/2012/07/endocrine-
disruption-and-whats-in.html

(11) Endocrine Disrupting Chemicals in Drinking
Water: Risks to Human Health and the
Environment. (2013, June 18). Retrieved
December 23, 2015, from
http://www.hhs.gov/asl/testify/2010/02/t20100225
a.html

(12) International Society of Indoor Air Quality and
Climate, Proceedings, 5th International Conference
on Indoor Air Quality and Climate: Indoor Air '90,
Toronto (Canada) 1990. (1990).

(13) Cancer Prevention Alert. (n.d.). Retrieved
December 23, 2015, from
http://www.preventcancer.com/press/pdfs/hazardo
us.pdf

(14) Mercola, MD, J. (2012, January 16). Beware:
Some Green Cleaning Products May Not Be Very
Green. Retrieved December 23, 2015, from

http://articles.mercola.com/sites/articles/archive/20
12/01/16/toxic-chemicals-in-green-cleaning-
products.aspx

(15) Household Products Database - Health and Safety
Information on Household Products. (n.d.).
Retrieved December 23, 2015, from
http://householdproducts.nlm.nih.gov/cgi-
bin/household/prodtree?prodcat=Inside the Home

(16) Winter, R. (2009). Introduction. In *A Consumer's
Dictionary of Cosmetic Ingredients* (7th ed., p. 1).
New York, New York: Three Rivers Press.

(17) Winter, R. (2009). Introduction. In *A Consumer's
Dictionary of Cosmetic Ingredients* (7th ed., p.3).
New York, New York: Three Rivers Press.

(18) Winter, R. (2009). Introduction. In *A Consumer's
Dictionary of Cosmetic Ingredients* (7th ed., p. 5).
New York, New York: Three Rivers Press.

(19) Darbre, P. (2005, September 1). Aluminum,
Antiperspirants and Breast Cancer. Retrieved
December 23, 2015, from
http://www.ncbi.nlm.nih.gov/pubmed/16045991

(20) Pope, G. (2004, February 1). Concentration of
Parabens in Human Breast Tumors. Retrieved
December 23, 2015, from
http://www.ncbi.nlm.nih.gov/pubmed/14745841

(21) Suzuki, D. (n.d.). 'Dirty Dozen' cosmetic
chemicals to avoid. Retrieved December 23, 2015,
from
http://www.davidsuzuki.org/issues/health/science/t
oxics/dirty-dozen-cosmetic-chemicals/

(22) Kaskey, J. (2015, March 20). Monsanto
Weedkiller is "Probably Carcinogenic" WHO says.
Retrieved December 23, 2015, from

(http://www.bloomberg.com/news/articles/2015-03-20/who-classifies-monsanto-s-glyphosate-as-probably-carcinogenic-)

(23) IARC Monographs Volume 112: Evaluation of five organophosphate insecticides and herbicides. (2015, March 20). Retrieved December 23, 2015, from https://www.iarc.fr/en/media-centre/iarcnews/pdf/MonographVolume112.pdf

(24) Glyphosate-based herbicides are toxic and endocrine disruptors in human cell lines. (2009, August 21). Retrieved December 23, 2015, from http://www.ncbi.nlm.nih.gov/pubmed/19539684

(25) Gasnier, C., Dumont, C., Benachour, N., Clair, E., Chagnon, M., & Séralini, G. (n.d.). Glyphosate-based herbicides are toxic and endocrine disruptors in human cell lines. *Toxicology,* 184-191.

(26) Mercola, MD, J. (n.d.). Monsanto: A Sustainable Ag Company? Retrieved December 23, 2015, from (http://articles.mercola.com/sites/articles/archive/2015/03/28/monsanto-sustainable-agriculture-company.aspx

(27) Kurenbach, B., Marjoshi, D., Amábile-Cuevas, C., Ferguson, G., Godsoe, W., Gibson, P., & Heinemann, J. (2015). Sublethal Exposure to Commercial Formulations of the Herbicides Dicamba, 2,4-Dichlorophenoxyacetic Acid, and Glyphosate Cause Changes in Antibiotic Susceptibility in Escherichia coli and Salmonella enterica serovar Typhimurium. *MBio.*

(28) Mercola, MD, J. (2009, October 10). Why are Monsanto Insiders Now Appointed to Protect Your Food Safety? Retrieved December 24, 2015, from http://articles.mercola.com/sites/articles/archive/20

09/10/10/Obama-Monsanto-Alliance-Too-Close-for-Comfort.aspx

(29) Lempert, P. (2004, July 21). Is your bottled water coming from a faucet? Retrieved December 24, 2015, from http://www.today.com/food/your-bottled-water-coming-faucet-2D80555502

(30) Chait, J. (2014, July 3). Can You Certify Organic Water? Retrieved December 24, 2015, from http://organic.about.com/od/organicindustrybasics/f/Can-You-Certify-Organic-Water.htm

(31) EWG's Shopper's Guide to Pesticides in Produce™. (n.d.). Retrieved December 24, 2015, from http://www.ewg.org/foodnews/summary.php

(32) Mercury Levels in Fish | NRDC. (n.d.). Retrieved December 24, 2015, from http://www.nrdc.org/health/effects/mercury/guide.asp

(33) Koff, A. (n.d.). What is the link between toxins in the body and weight loss? - Weight Loss. Retrieved December 24, 2015, from https://www.sharecare.com/health/weight-loss/what-link-between-toxins-weight

(34) Arsenic, cadmium, lead, and mercury in sweat: A systematic review. (2012, February 22). Retrieved December 24, 2015, from http://www.ncbi.nlm.nih.gov/pubmed/22505948?utm_source=Clean Newsletter&utm_campaign=1e67e6ca60-sweating__8_10_2015&utm_medium=email&utm_term=0_88ac180814-1e67e6ca60-399782405&mc_cid=1e67e6ca60&mc_eid=02bad8d471

(35) Human excretion of bisphenol A: Blood, urine, and sweat (BUS) study. (2011, December 27). Retrieved December 24, 2015, from http://www.ncbi.nlm.nih.gov/pubmed/22253637?u tm_source=Clean Newsletter&utm_campaign=1e67e6ca60-sweating__8_10_2015&utm_medium=email&utm _term=0_88ac180814-1e67e6ca60-399782405&mc_cid=1e67e6ca60&mc_eid=02bad 8d471

(36) Mercola, MD, J. (2008, October 14). Talcum Powder Linked to Ovarian Cancer. Retrieved December 24, 2015, from http://articles.mercola.com/sites/articles/archive/20 08/10/14/talcum-powder-linked-to-ovarian-cancer.aspx#!

(37) What's In a Cigarette? (n.d.). Retrieved December 24, 2015, from http://www.lung.org/stop-smoking/smoking-facts/whats-in-a-cigarette.html?referrer=https://www.google.com/

(38) Elkhaim, Y. (2013, September 13). The Truth About How Much Water You Should Really Drink. Retrieved December 24, 2015, from http://health.usnews.com/health-news/blogs/eat-run/2013/09/13/the-truth-about-how-much-water-you-should-really-drink

(39) Urinary Tract Infection (UTI) Prevention. (2012, February 7). Retrieved December 24, 2015, from https://www.healthstatus.com/health_blog/ovulatio n-2/urinary-tract-infection-uti-prevention/

(40) Mercola, MD, J. (2013, February 14). What You See in the Toilet Says Something About Your Health. Retrieved December 24, 2015, from

http://articles.mercola.com/sites/articles/archive/20
13/02/14/normal-stool.aspx

(41) Hart, A. (2014, January 5). Is there castoreum in
your nondairy milk substitute beverage? Retrieved
December 26, 2015, from
http://www.examiner.com/article/is-there-
castoreum-your-nondairy-milk-substitute-beverage

(42) Winter, R(2009) A Consumer's Dictionary of
Cosmetic Ingredients. Three Rivers Press 7th ed
pg. 138

(43) Edelson, MD, S., & Mitchell, D. (2003). The
Role of Environmental Toxins in the Autoimmune
Process. In What Your Doctor May Not Tell You
About Autoimmune Disorders: The Revolutionary,
Drug-Free Treatments for Thyroid Disease, Lupus,
MS, IBD, Chronic Fatigue; Rheumatoid Arthritis,
and Other Diseases. Mount Pocono, PA: Grand
Central Publishing; The Hatchett Book Group.

(44) Skin Deep® Cosmetics Database | EWG. (n.d.).
Retrieved January 18, 2016, from
http://www.ewg.org/skindeep/

(45) Kolpin, D., Blazer, V., Gray, J., Focazio, M.,
Young, J., Alvarez, D., . . . Barber, L. (2012).
Chemical contaminants in water and sediment near
fish nesting sites in the Potomac River basin:
Determining potential exposures to smallmouth
bass (Micropterus dolomieu). Science of The Total
Environment, 443, 700-716. doi:doi:10.1016

(46) Ganim, S., & Tran, L. (2016, January 13). How tap water became toxic in Flint, Michigan - CNN.com. Retrieved January 22, 2016, from http://www.cnn.com/2016/01/11/health/toxic-tap-water-flint-michigan/

(47) Karimi, F. (2016, January 25). Sebring, Ohio: Schools closed as water tests demanded - CNN.com. Retrieved January 25, 2016, from http://www.cnn.com/2016/01/25/us/sebring-lead-water-investigation/

(48) LaMotte, S. (2016, January 21). How to test for lead in your home water supply - CNN.com. Retrieved January 25, 2016, from http://www.cnn.com/2016/01/21/health/lead-testing-home-drinking-water/

(49) Organic Foods: All You Need to Know. (2016, January). Retrieved January 27, 2016, from http://www.helpguide.org/articles/healthy-eating/organic-foods.htm

(50) 12 things you should know about common pain relievers. (n.d.). Retrieved January 27, 2016, from http://www.health.harvard.edu/pain/12-things-you-should-know-about-pain-relievers

(51) Zucchini, Fennel & White Bean Pasta. (n.d.). Retrieved January 27, 2016, from http://www.eatingwell.com/recipes/zucchini_fennel_bean_pasta.html

(52) Turmeric Rice Recipe - Food.com. (n.d.). Retrieved January 27, 2016, from http://www.food.com/recipe/turmeric-rice-48162

(53) Other Uses of Petroleum. (n.d.). Retrieved January 27, 2016, from

http://www.petroleum.co.uk/other-uses-of-petroleum

(54) Cauliflower with Garlic Sauce. (n.d.). Retrieved January 27, 2016, from http://www.davita.com/recipes/vegetables/cauliflower-with-garlic-sauce/r/5018

(55) H. (n.d.). Soluble Fiber ~ The Irritable Bowel Syndrome Good Foods. Retrieved January 27, 2016, from http://www.helpforibs.com/diet/fiber1.asp

(56) Cans without BPA. (n.d.). Retrieved January 27, 2016, from http://www.inspirationgreen.com/bpa-lined-cans.html

(57) B. M. (2013, March 25). Publisher's Platform: Mike Taylor and the Myth of Monsanto's Man | Food Safety News. Retrieved January 29, 2016, from http://www.foodsafetynews.com/2013/03/publishers-platform-mike-taylor-and-the-myth-of-monsantos-man/#.Vqu5HCvF_Uk

(58) J. M. (2014, November 4). Neonicotinoid Pesticides Are Too Toxic to Use. Retrieved January 29, 2016, from http://articles.mercola.com/sites/articles/archive/2014/11/04/neonicotinoid-pesticide-use.aspx

(59) J. M. (2009, November 21). France Finds Monsanto Guilty of Lying. Retrieved January 30, 2016, from http://articles.mercola.com/sites/articles/archive/2009/11/21/france-finds-monsanto-guilty-of-lying.aspx

(60) J. M. (2009, March 7). Monsantos Many Attempts to Destroy All Seeds but Their Own.

Retrieved January 30, 2016, from
http://articles.mercola.com/sites/articles/archive/20
09/03/07/Monsantos-Many-Attempts-to-Destroy-
All-Seeds-but-Their-Own.aspx

(61) Seneff, S. (2015, August 19). Stephanie Seneff,
PhD on Glyphosate (RoundUp) Poisoning.
Retrieved February 05, 2016, from
https://www.youtube.com/watch?v=qYC6oyBglZI

Index

Printed in Dunstable, United Kingdom